People ask me: What kind of Native healer are you? You think they would know by my name, but I guess most people don't know the Native spiritual ways anymore. I am a Grizzlybear doctor. That means that my primary power and gift is from the grizzlybear, but he is connected to other things such as the Sun and Moon, lightning and thunder, deer and wolves, ravens, hawks, and eagles, snakes and rocks, water and fish, wind and rain, and many other relations in Nature.

My training was determined by the Great Creator, the spirits, the ancestors, and the elders. I started out as a dreamer, became an herbalist, then a seer and visionary, later a healer, and eventually evolved into a spiritual doctor. Essentially this means I see the spirits, hear the spirits, work with the spirits, and they work through me.

NATIVE HEALER

The path to an ancient healing art

▼   ▼   ▼   ▼   ▼

MEDICINE GRIZZLYBEAR LAKE

HarperPaperbacks
A Division of HarperCollins*Publishers*

HarperPaperbacks *A Division of* HarperCollins*Publishers*
10 East 53rd Street, New York, N.Y. 10022

A previous edition of this book was published in 1991 by Quest Books, a division of The Theosophical Publishing House.

Cover photograph courtesy of the National Museum of the American Indian/Smithsonian Institution #4771

First HarperPaperbacks printing: August 1993

Printed in the United States of America

HarperPaperbacks and colophon are trademarks of HarperCollins*Publishers*

10 9 8 7 6 5 4 3 2 1

I dedicate this book to my wife, Tela Starhawk, to my children, to my brother Ron, and to the many Elders who have taught and trained me to serve our people.

It takes a lot of time, effort, resources and funds to sponsor Sacred Sun Dancers. Tela and I have been donating a portion of our publishing royalties toward these dances, and if you the general public would like to help, please send donations to:

Gilbert Brady
Hereditary Sun Dance Chief,
For the Crazy Dog Society
of Northern Cheyenne Nation
P.O. Box 155
Lame Deer, MT 59043

or

Charles Chips
Hereditary Lakota Sun Dance Chief
P.O. Box 257
Wanblee, SD 57577

CONTENTS

Foreword by Rolling Thunder, ix
Foreword by Charlie Thom, xi
Acknowledgments, xv
Preface, xvii
Introduction, 1
1. Becoming a Native Healer, 7
2. Trials and Tests, 16
3. Power Dreams, 30
4. Vision Seeking and Power Quests, 47
5. The Calling, 66
6. The Training of Women Healers:
   Present and Past, 86
7. Apprenticeship, 115
8. Native Healing:
   Its Philosophy and Practice, 124
9. Psychic Phenomena and Symbolism
   in Native Healing, 138
10. Plant People, 157
11. The Medicine Sweat, 166
12. Native Practices for Healing Yourself, 190
13. The Native Healer in Today's Society, 200
    Epilogue, 213
    Appendix: Spiritual Violations, 215

FOREWORD

rolling thunder

▼   ▼   ▼   ▼   ▼   ▼

I HAVE KNOWN BOBBY LAKE, WHOSE NATIVE NAME IS Medicine Grizzlybear, for approximately twenty years. He was one of my apprentices, and I am proud to wholeheartedly endorse this book.

Bobby was taught and trained by over sixteen different elderly medicine men and women and traditional ceremonial leaders from different tribes. Rarely do you find novices being honored with that many mentors and diversity, either in the past or in the present. As I stated in one of my previous letters of support on his behalf when he worked at the University: "Bobby is a recipient of rare and sacred knowledge, a young but wise traditional Native healer, a genuine shaman of the highest degree, and a real asset to our new generation . . . what he offers will serve to be a real contribution to all mankind, and especially our Native people."

Thus, in this book is a rare opportunity for both the public and the professional to learn about shamanism from somebody who has been taught, trained, studied and practiced in both worlds and societies. I therefore highly recommend it with prayers that it will be a success in terms of publication, and prove to be of value to those in search of New Age and future-oriented forms of knowledge.

Rolling Thunder
Intertribal Medicine Man
Carlin, Nevada

FOREWORD

charlie thom

▼   ▼   ▼   ▼   ▼   ▼

MEDICINE MEN AND WOMEN ARE AN ENDANGERED SPECIES. For many tribes the role and function of medicine man has already become extinct. The crazy and rapid advancement of technology, science, medicine, and Western way of thinking is putting the rest of us on the verge of extinction. We cannot survive without our sacred mountains, ceremonial grounds, holy places, and subsistence areas. We need the places that the Great Creator gave us in the Beginning in order to seek visions and guidance, acquire power and knowledge, conduct sacred rituals and ceremonies, and to gather our herbs and spirits for healing. As civilization expands it encroaches upon, desecrates, and destroys the natural resources that we as natural healers need in order to make the people healthy and well.

Our powers come from our relations in Nature. They are our advisers and allies. Their hides, claws, furs, teeth, and feathers are our spiritual tools. These are the powers we use for healing, ritual, ceremony, and to help keep the world in balance. We are keepers of the land, we have the ancient knowledge and future vision to help modern people survive and continue as a species. We will not be able to save this Earth if our natural sources of power and knowledge continue to be destroyed.

There were certain mountains on this continent where we could privately visit with the Creator and his spirits. Now he no longer comes to these places because modern people, of all races, have either polluted or destroyed them. There were secret healing waters, springs, and ceremonial grounds where one could go to be miraculously healed, as if by magic, but it was not magic. It was a real source of sacred and natural power put here on this Earth for that purpose; and now these places are totally destroyed.

Medicine men and women were highly respected in the old days. Theirs was a sacred profession, and they served a special role that very few people could qualify for. And there were many different roles a medicine man could fulfill; some were priestly, others were doctoring, and some were a combination of both. For example, there were ritual performers and ceremonial leaders, dreamers, seers, trance doctors, healers, and sucking doctors. All of the roles were medico-religious, and spiritual in nature. The tribe took good care of medicine men and women, and they cared for the people, to the point of taking on their pain, problems, illnesses, and injuries; they would even die for them if necessary.

A medicine man or woman today is much different from the ones in the past. It is more difficult for a medicine man or woman today to survive and help the people, and it will be more so in the future. It takes a special kind of species to carry on the elite system. And that is what makes Medicine Grizzlybear, one of my former apprentices, so special. He was taught and trained by sixteen different elderly medicine men/women from different tribes. The voices of the ancestors therefore speak through him. What he has to offer in this book is a rare opportunity for the people to learn high spiritual knowledge, the kind that can only come from a medicine man who has trained on the highest spiritual mountain.

Charlie Thom
Karuk Medicine Man and Ceremonial Leader
Mt. Shasta, California

ACKNOWLEDGMENTS

▼ ▼ ▼ ▼ ▼ ▼

I GIVE SPECIAL THANKS TO KAY KENNEDY FOR ENCOURAG-
ing me to write this book. I also want to thank Shirley
Nicholson, its editor, for her professional expertise
and dedication in making the manuscript become a
success.

I wish to thank the following for permission to
publish their material: The Lowie Museum of An-
thropology, University of California at Berkeley for
the account of Fanny Flounder's initiation ceremony,
which first appeared in a study by Spott and Kroeber,
1946.

▼ ▼ ▼ ▼ ▼ ▼

THIS BOOK IS A RESULT OF INFORMATION I HAVE BEEN DEAL-
ing with during my twenty years of apprenticeship
and practice as a traditional Native healer and ceremonial leader, or what Western professionals call a
"shaman." I have published most of this information
in a number of journals and well-known New Age
magazines. What is presented here is an update and
synthesis of the concepts, theories, and applications I
have been sharing with Native communities, professional audiences, and the public via conferences,
training workshops, lectures, and seminars.

Throughout the text you will see the words "medicine man or woman," "shaman," "Indian doctor,"

and "Native healer" being used interchangeably. This is in order to relate to a larger audience and to the many different perspectives and definitions of the terms. Personally, I prefer to say "Native healer," which is more in keeping with the cultural perspective. The word "shaman" or "medicine man" is not indigenous. Secondly, the concept and role of a shaman is often associated with sorcery, which is diametrically opposed to that of the healer, while the role and function of a medicine man or woman has often been applied in a general way to include those who perform more priestly functions. The traditional Native healer, however, normally has a multifaceted role which includes training, knowledge, power, and ability to serve in a number of medico-religious functions, such as herbalist, seer, ceremonial leader, doctor, and spiritual teacher. But even here there are degrees of development, function, and sometimes specialization. As understood and defined from the Native perspective, the Native healer is a combination of several roles and functions comparable to that of a physician, psychologist, priest, teacher, and mystic, all rolled up into one.

INTRODUCTION

▼   ▼   ▼   ▼   ▼   ▼

TRADITIONAL NATIVE HEALERS WERE THE PEOPLE WHO PRO-
vided medical leadership for the community in the
past, for most Native tribal systems. They were the
seers, visionaries, doctors, and counselors for the people. They advised the people about good health practices which were medico-religious in nature, and they
taught them how to develop spiritually. When the
people became sick, the Native healer doctored them.
And if the healer did not have an answer to a particular problem, he or she would seek a vision by consult-
ing with the Great Creator and spirits to find solutions. During such times the shaman could often see
into the future. In some ways, that is what I am trying
to share here.

The traditional Native healer is an endangered species now. But there is an opportunity for modern Native and Western people to share in the knowledge of past Native healers and the few remaining ones who are with us in the New Age.

Native shamans were and still are "natural practitioners." They use natural knowledge, natural methods, and Nature in order to doctor a patient. Their training and development is very difficult. It usually starts with a dream, followed by a mystical experience of enlightenment, an illness, an accident, a disease, or even a death experience. They do not learn from textbooks; they do not get their knowledge from attending college; and they do not get their experience from experimenting on animals or humans. They do, however, undergo an extensive apprenticeship and training which is rigorous, full of suffering and sacrifice, new challenge, and new learning. In order to qualify to heal others, they first must learn to overcome and heal their own sickness, problem, injury, or disease.

Contrary to modern Western misconceptions, shamanism or Native healing is a complex system of learning far removed from the field of magic and quackery. It may not be like Western standards of preparation, but in its own way it is very stringent and demanding. The novice must study new bodies of knowledge in the form of myths and prayer formulas, each designed for a different kind of sickness, disease, ailment, or injury, including death-related phenomena. During an apprenticeship the novice studies the elderly shaman's philosophy, expertise, methods, and approaches to healing. At this time he or she is under strict supervision. In some situations the entire process might start all over again due to a new dream, vision, pain, or psychic-mystical experience. Such a new occurrence provides the apprentice with an opportunity to gain more diversified knowledge, skills, and experience; it also provides him or her with depth and breadth in the profession.

Native healers use "spiritual" power in healing. They get this power from a number of sources: from the Great Spirit, from within themselves, from the spiritual and physical forces and powers in Nature. An example of a spirit might be the ghost of a deceased relative who was a shaman, or it could be a certain spirit that lives in a mountain. Sources of power might include physical entities such as the power of the Raven, Hawk, Eagle, Bear, Wolf, Coyote, Deer, Salmon, a Bug, a two-headed Snake, or the sweat lodge, a waterfall, wind, lightning and thunder, a star, the Moon or Sun. All things in Nature, seen and unseen, are considered a source of spiritual power which certain Native healers might be connected to and use in healing.

The shaman's power might come from one source in Nature or numerous sources. All such sources are considered the Great Creator's helpers. Native healers use these powers, as a means to diagnose and cure physical, mental, emotional, and spiritual illnesses. They also use these powers for self-protection, self-guidance, self-development, and they attempt to apply the same to their patients.

The Hawk is not just a beautiful bird who has certain physical characteristics; it is a spiritual source of power. It can be used for seeing because it is a good seer; it can be used for protection because it is a strong fighter; it can be used for soul travel because it can fly long distance against great odds and the forces of nature. The Bear is a doctor because it is wise, lives in the wilderness, has human-like qualities, digs for roots, and knows exactly what kinds of herbs to use in healing a wide variety of illnesses, including arthritis, broken bones, and injuries. The Hummingbird is a strong doctor for mental illnesses because it uses color, sound, and vibration in healing. It is fast enough to catch up to your lost mind and bring it back and put it in balance with your brain and body. The Flickerbird works with fire; it can heal burns, take away fevers, and eat the bugs (diseases) out of your system. The Wolf is a scout and can track down the cause of illness. It is a strong protector and it can fend off evil entities while protecting the patient during the time of healing with other spiritual powers. The wind can blow away sickness, the clouds can be used as purifiers, the fog as a protector, the water as a purifier, and any number of different plants and trees as healing agents, helping both physically and spiritually. The Snake can go into the body and trace down the source of illness and devour it.

The Native healer has been trained to know about these powers and how to use them in healing. The powers are symbolically reflected as tools of the trade the Native doctor uses. For example, a medicine man might wear a bear hide or a wolf hide and use an eagle wing fan or flicker feathers while dancing and singing over the patient. When he does this, he becomes that power; that power works through him. They become one in the healing process. So the regalia you see the Native doctor use are not simply "fetishes" for magic and trickery; they are actual physical and spiritual power "tools of the trade" being employed in much the same way a modern physician uses a stethoscope, X-ray machine, ultrasound, or lab tests.

In some ways, the power being used defines what kind of Indian doctor, medicine man or woman, or Native healer one is. There are several kinds. A trance doctor goes into altered states of consciousness or soul-travels, but mostly uses his or her own mental powers to diagnose and cure illness. A sucking doctor uses certain powers from Nature to diagnose the sickness and suck the pain or poison out of a patient. A hand-healer normally uses innate powers of healing, the power of the Great Creator, and certain powers in Nature to doctor the patient. A spiritual doctor uses a variety of spirits and powers, including all of the above, to diagnose, protect and heal the patient. Native healers might specialize in a particular kind of healing. Native female practitioners focus on illnesses related to menses, menopause, and childbirth. Others specialize in mental-emotional problems related to stress and sorcery. Some might handle a variety of illnesses. Among the northwest California tribes I would be considered a "sucking doctor and spiritual doctor"; the plains people would consider me a Grizzlybear doctor.

The following chapters will attempt to help you understand this complex system of knowledge and application a little better.

1 ▾ BECOMING A NATIVE HEALER

▾   ▾   ▾   ▾   ▾   ▾

YOU DON'T JUST WAKE UP ONE MORNING AND SAY, "GEE, I would like to be a medicine man." It doesn't work that way. There is something different about a person who is meant to be a Native healer. You are born with a special kind of power, gift, talent, and knowledge. It is not your power; it belongs to the Great Creator and the people. It is only loaned to you. And it must be handled in the right and proper way or someone could get hurt.

I have never stood up in front of a group of people and said, "I am a medicine man." I rarely talk about it. If the people are meant to know, they will know. But there have been times, when someone pushed it far enough, that I would say; "Yes, I am a servant of the Great Creator. I am a traditional Native healer, spiritual teacher, and ceremonial leader." It is said that way because of humbleness, not out of shame, not out of boasting, but due to reality. I say it that way because that is what the Great Creator, the spirits, and my elderly mentors have told me I am. If the people want to call me a medicine man, I am honored. But a real medicine man should not have to identify himself as such. It is not the Indian way.

I don't fit most people's stereotype of what a Native healer should be. I am not a wise old man living in a remote part of the reservation in poverty, waiting to be discovered by an anthropologist or writer or some kind of psychic researcher. I am not a full-blooded Indian. I am not tall and dark skinned with a big nose. In fact, I don't even fit the description of my name, Medicine Grizzlybear. My friend Archie Fire Lamedeer should probably have that name because he is about 6 feet, 3 inches tall, weighs 240 pounds, and is big like a grizzly. He even has the silver streaks and dark coloring. We laugh about it because we "know" that each medicine man or woman has a special name that the Great Creator gives him or her. Sometimes that name is kept secret. I kept my name secret for over a decade. Archie Lamedeer has a secret name. Martin High Bear, another friend who is also a well-known medicine man, has a special name—Rocky Boy. He has this name because he works with the power and spirit of the rock people. Such names have power. They really mean something because they are your password, as a Native healer, to the Great Creator, the spirits, and the Mother Earth. And with the name comes responsibility.

So I didn't just wake up one morning and decide to pick a name that would make me more Indian. I earned it by fasting, sweating, and through a ten-day vision quest on a sacred mountain top. I didn't pick my name; I didn't pick the powers that go with the name; and I didn't really pick this profession. It was given to me in an honorable and clean way. I didn't want to be a Native healer—I was chosen for it. Four different times in my life I went to elderly medicine people in the Indian way and asked them to take it out of me. I gave them a lot of money, gifts, and even offered hard labor to have the power taken away. I didn't want the responsibility, hardship, sacrifice, and strict life that went with it. Two of these Elders refused. One tried to do what I asked and died exactly a year later. The fourth one, Rolling Thunder, really scolded me. He said: "This is not your choosing. You don't have the right or authority to interfere with what the Great Spirit has decided. You were chosen to be a medicine man long before you came into this body on this Earth. You have a duty and responsibility to follow the calling. If not, you will hurt your family, your people, and the spiritual function and design of the Universe. Sure, it's a tough life. Your own Indian people will make fun of you, they will talk bad about you, they will probably even call you a phony or something. But the Great Creator knows, the Mother Earth knows, your relations in Nature know, the numerous people from all walks of life you will heal, help, and teach will know; and you will know. That is all that really matters. And when things get tough in your life, you'll just have to grin and bear it. That is one of the ways for a true medicine man. You take on the suffering, the fear, the hate, the anger, the pain, the confusion, and the sickness of the people. That is why you are different. And you can't run and hide from it. You were put here on the Earth to do a job for the Great Creator. Like it or not, you've got to be strong and just do it."

In the olden days, the elderly people usually knew ahead of time when a Native healer was coming to the tribe. They would know through dreams, signs, omens, and ceremony. Sometimes they would know before the child was born; at other times they would find out at its birth. Sometimes, however, they didn't find out until the child was growing up. It all depended on the tribal custom, belief, ways, and degree of spiritual evolvement. Nowadays very few people know about these things. The Native tribes that are more traditional in their life-style will have a way of knowing, but the more assimilated tribes and Christian indoctrinated tribal societies don't even care. For some of these tribes the role and function of a medicine person has become extinct, a thing of the past.

One of my elderly mentors was from the Iroquois Six Nations. I stem from the Iroquois Six Nations Natives, but I was mainly taught and trained by the Yurok and Karuk in northwestern California. This mentor told me he knew about me when I was still a child. He said he dreamt about me, that a bear came and told him. Although I met this Native healer when I was younger, I didn't really get to study and train under him until I was in my late twenties. His name was Beeman Logan, a hereditary Seneca chief and medicine man. Another great chief said he knew I would come to him some day. He said he hoped I would come before he got old and died. His name was Chief Harry Watt. He died two years after I finally got to see him, and he helped put me up on Seneca mountain. I had to go 3000 miles back home, from California to New York, to do that. It was like a salmon going back home to its original birthplace to spawn and die. Chief Harry Watt said he knew that a young man in his tribe would inherit the medicine power and return to his people; but he said also he felt sad that the people would not be ready for this person. He was right.

Evidently, the day I was born something strange happened. Thunder and lightning cracked all over the Six Nations mountains and Seneca territory; some said it was a freak hailstorm with hailstones the size of baseballs. This also happened each time I died. Four times so far in my life I have been pronounced dead. Two other times I know I died, but no one except my wife was around to verify it. Of course I was only dead a short time, but being dead is dead, whether temporary or permanent. I know that when I get old and finally die that there will be a bad storm, much worse than the others, because I have already seen it in a vision. More than likely, though, the people won't even notice it; they won't understand what such events mean.

The path to becoming a Native healer is full of trials and tribulations, suffering and sacrifice. It encompasses all facets of life and of human nature. It involves the physical and spiritual, the mental and emotional. Along this path are certain stages.

The way I understand it, these include: 1) inheritance—you are born with the potentiality genetically; 2) the calling, which usually comes in the form of a dream or a series of dreams; 3) the initiation, which occurs via an illness, disease, accident, injury, sometimes a severe mental or emotional problem, or a profound psychic or mystical experience, or a death experience; 4) the vision quest and spiritual training when one is guided to a specific power center in Nature to acquire and activate power; 5) the evaluation and confirmation by the elders, and the apprenticeship; 6) the actual practice of being a Native healer, which in itself is a never-ending learning process because the neophyte or his or her family members frequently become ill. Although it seems very unfair, this strange relationship with "power" and encounters with new illnesses serve as the basis for native healers to gain new experiences and knowledge. Unfortunately, sometimes they lose a patient or even a family member, but this is how it has been cosmically designed for healers to learn.

People ask me: What kind of Native healer are you? You think they would know by my name, but I guess most people don't know the Native spiritual ways anymore. I am a Grizzlybear doctor. That means that my primary power and gift is from the grizzlybear, but he is connected to other things such as the Sun and Moon, lightning and thunder, mountains and rivers, hummingbirds and plants, deer and wolves, ravens, hawks, and eagles, snakes and rocks, water and fish, wind and rain, and many other relations in Nature. Though among the northwestern California tribes I would be considered a "sucking doctor and spiritual doctor," other tribal groups such as the plains, southwest, and Alaskan would consider me a "Bear doctor."

My training was determined by the Great Creator, the spirits, the ancestors, and the Elders. I started out as a dreamer, became an herbalist, then a seer and visionary, later a healer, and eventually evolved into a spiritual doctor. Essentially this means that I see the spirits, hear the spirits, work with the spirits, and they work through me. I am not a trance doctor, however; I do not go into a trance. I was also taught to use the sacred sweat lodge for ceremony and doctoring, and the War Dance Ceremony was willed to me. I am not a "pipe carrier" as I did not start out in that kind of tribal system. My own Iroquois people might not even recognize me for what I really am because for the last 200 years or so, we have not had individual medicine men and women. Instead we have societies who do the doctoring, such as the False Face Society and the Little Water Society. Originally we had Native healers but that changed according to need. In the last decade a few individual medicine men have emerged, such as Mad Bear Anderson and Beeman Logan, and they were criticized by their own people for breaking the norm.

Maybe the people need to relearn that it is not they who have the authority to choose or decide who will be a medicine man; the Great Creator makes this kind of decision. My record is straight with the Great Creator despite anyone's judgment. It has to be straight in order to qualify for the knowledge and powers, and to be his servant. I don't claim to be a saint, and I surely don't want to be anyone's guru. But I have strived to be a higher spiritual person. I wanted to be spiritual because I had good mentors to emulate. And the mountains do that to a person. The spirits of the mountains are magical and mysterious. They pull a person like a magnet. We need mountains as symbols of spirituality and reminders of sacredness. Every human being who walks the earth should be inclined toward spiritual development and evolvement because in the Beginning we were spirits. Perhaps most people have forgotten that reality since they have become civilized humans. Maybe they have forgotten that we are still spirits in a human shell.

So it is with the makeup of our entire being. We have a mind, a body, and a soul, and we all have spiritual guardians of some kind. From the moment we entered this earth plane we had to have assistance; we could not have possibly made it on our own. And when we die and leave these bodies, our guardian spirit will help us to the other side, into the spirit world. However, sometimes it happens that we make so many violations upon this earth that our guardian spirit deserts us out of disgust, or a sorcerer or an evil spirit takes it away.

That guardian spirit or ally is real. It is an archetypal part of our unconscious, and for most it will take on some kind of animal form. According to the Law of Cosmic Duality there are two sides to everything. We are human, and we are also animal. Through the vision quest we find out what our animal spirit power is or can become. Sometimes a life crisis, accident, sickness, or disease will bring this side of ourselves to the surface. When this happens, we need to confront it, become one with it, and cultivate it. This is another reason our Native people have the sacred sweat lodge and vision quest. They are the spiritual tools we were given to find out who we really are and to evolve higher spiritually. I have met people who claim they identified their "totem" through meditation or a tarot card reading, but they are only fooling themselves. There are many different kinds of symbols—animals, spirits, even demons and phantoms—in our subconscious mind. There is no easy way out in the process of "self-discovery," and all races of humankind have had the process of fasting and vision-seeking in order to get in touch with their real Self or what some have called "higher self."

2 ▼ TRIALS AND TESTS

▼   ▼   ▼   ▼   ▼   ▼

THERE IS A PREDETERMINED PATH THAT ONE MUST FOLLOW in order to become a Native healer, or medicine person. You are born with the power, you inherit the power, or it can be willed to you. Then you have the calling. Most Native healers are therefore bloodline; their parents, grandparents, or foreparents were medicine people. In this way it is passed down through the genetic and psychic structure. But even if you are born with it, you will not necessarily "become." Sometimes it passes over a generation or two and resurfaces, as with artists in a family. All of the children of an artist will inherit some degree of artistic talent or ability, but as the generations go by the family might not notice it. Sometime later, one of the grandchildren might suddenly display talent and the people say, "She's just like her grandmother (or great-grandfather)!" Medicine power is the same way only more complex and more difficult. It is extremely hard to explain to people who have never lived the Indian way or been raised in that cultural context.

Even if you have the capacity, the path to becoming a Native healer is not easy. There is evidently some kind of definite cosmic procedure that we must follow. You can't go to college and study for it. It is not like training to become a doctor in the White man's way. There are no books, no units of credit. But you do have tests and exams to pass. It is only through severe pain, suffering, sickness, and death itself that you gain access to another form of reality. That "other world" is where you find the knowledge, experience, qualifications, and power to help the people.

The calling comes in the form of a dream, accident, sickness, injury, disease, near-death experience, or even actual death. For example, when I was four years old my family took me on a picnic up in the Six Nations area of the Allegheny Mountains, outside of Salamanca, New York, near a place known as Thunder Rocks. I can still remember it clearly, although I was very young at the time. I had been complaining of a sore throat, headache, fever, and leg cramps, and the long drive in the car from Buffalo made my illness worse. I didn't have anyone to play with since my younger brother was barely walking at the time. Although I was sick, I kept wishing I had other kids to play with. I don't know if it was my imagination or not, but I began to see little Indian people, much smaller than my younger brother. They were running around, dodging in and out behind trees, bushes, and rocks. I thought they were playing "peek-a-boo" with me. As sick as I was, I couldn't help laughing. As I played with them, they kept leading me farther and farther away from the picnic site. I got dizzy from all the running and playing around, and began to throw up. I don't remember much after that except that the little people kept pulling on me to get me up to go with them.

When I woke up I was in my bedroom at home in Tondawanda. My whole body was on fire with fever. The room was dark except for the abrupt flashing of lightning, the loud crack of thunder, and big balls of hailstones and rain hitting the window.

I saw a spirit standing at the foot of my bed, and it scared me. At first I thought it must be a dream, but it wasn't; everything around me was real. I'll never forget what that spirit looked like and how he was dressed. He wore a traditional Iroquois hat with one eagle feather sticking up on top and a sash made from hummingbird feathers strung across his shoulder. His long white hair dangled past his bearclaw necklace, and he held two items in his hand—an eaglewing fan and a small pipe. As I sat there shivering in amazement, he came closer and said; "Do not be afraid, my son. I am one of your ancestors. Watch what I do, as I sing and dance around you. And remember this, because someday when you get older you will help heal others the same way."

He blew smoke on me four times from his pipe. Then he brushed my body four times with the eaglewing feathers, as if catching something unseen and throwing it away. He put his hands on my forehead, chest, stomach and legs. Each time he growled like a bear, sang a very soft song, then slung his hands out toward the window.

The lightning and thunder got louder, and I became terrified. Hail suddenly broke through the glass window, and rain, hail, and wind rushed into my room with a mighty force. It blew right through the old man spirit. He reached toward the window and gathered up rainwater with cupped hands. Then he walked over to me and sprinkled it all over my head. I could actually see a horrible black thing leave my body, followed by streaks of fire. It was sucked out through the window and never returned.

I started hollering in fear. I didn't understand what was going on. All I wanted was my mother. She came running into the room, turned on the light, and looked at all the wet mess on my bed and around the room. Then she fell down on my bed crying: "Oh my God, he is alive! He is alive! Doctor, come here quick. He is not dead after all! Look, he is alive!"

I was sick and bedridden for about a week. I found out when I got older that I had been pronounced dead, and my parents were just waiting for the ambulance to take my body away. I was diagnosed as having rheumatic fever, polio, and pneumonia, and my fever had shot over 106 degrees. Evidently I had been lost in the woods for four days before anyone found me.

I was nine years old the second time I died. We had gone camping with my uncle Earl Blankenship and his family on the Cherokee reservation, beside a large creek or small river with a small lake nearby. My cousin and I went swimming, and he kept trying to wrestle with the other kids and dunk them under the water to scare them. After a while nobody would play with him, so he decided to get attention by starting a contest to see who could dive under the water and hold their breath the longest. He grabbed me and pulled me under. I tried to fight him off, but kept losing my breath. Then he must have gotten a cramp in his leg because he kept hollering, "My leg hurts and I can't swim." As he began to sink, he tried to use me as a prop and kept pushing me under while he tried to keep his head above water and gasp for air. I began to panic. I couldn't hold my breath any longer, and I couldn't get away from his deadly and desperate grip.

Next thing I knew the whole world turned black. I found myself going deeper and deeper into an abyss of darkness. One part of me could feel the heaviness of water all around, but another part felt total lightness. It was as if I had been caught in a whirlpool, some kind of funnel, where I could see light at the top but the bottom was narrow, dark, and swirling. I desperately fought for my life while being pulled down into a cold vacuum.

Then a calmness came over me, followed by warmth. I could hear Indian songs in the distance. The songs seemed to come closer. I found myself standing in an earthlodge type structure. In the middle was a fire pit surrounded by large poles, and in the shadows a group of people was singing. Different birds and masks were hung on the lodge poles— Raven, Wolf, and some masks that had long gray hair. The room was filled with smoke and the smell of cedar burning. A man and a woman, elderly Natives, walked out of the darkness into the light. They were so radiant that they blocked out the red colors of the sacred fire. The woman had turtle shell rattles on her legs, and when she danced I went into a trance. The elderly man had a turtle shell rattle in his hand, and he was naked except for a breechcloth. His face was painted in red and white stripes, a bearclaw necklace hung from his neck, yellow lightning designs were painted on his arms. The lightning streaks on his arms flashed as he reached for a bear hide and put it over his head. He no longer looked human but like a bear.

The elderly woman picked up a bowl obviously filled with hot water. She sprinkled some kind of herb into it and stirred it slowly, while singing. Her long braided white hair hung below her hips.

It was as if a magnet pulled me toward them as I walked over to the fire. They turned toward me and said: "You are not meant to be here, it is not your time yet. Here, sit down upon the ground and drink this tea." As I drank, they sang. The singing got louder as others I could not see in the shadows began to join in. The elderly man danced around me growling like a bear. He scratched my arms, chest, and legs with bear claws to the point that blood started to run from the small gashes.

The smoke-filled room made me drowsy, and I started to fall asleep. The last thing I remember from this dream was the old man saying: "We are your people, you have visited the medicine lodge. Someday you will be doing this for other people, so remember these songs. Here, take this basket of herbs, water, turtle shell rattle, bear claws and hide, and these sacred feathers. Whenever you need our help just smoke this pipe, call our names, and the Raven will bring you here again." The rattle and hypnotic rhythm of a turtle shell slowly drifted away, and my whole world was filled with light.

I don't really know how long I was under the water. The sun was at its apex in the sky, almost blinding, but a marvelous sight for someone who had just come back from the land of the dead (or was it just a dream?). A group of people crowded around. Somebody grabbed me and started squeezing my rib cage until I began to throw up. Someone else gave me mouth-to-mouth resuscitation. This went on for quite some time until I finally regained consciousness and a sense of what was going on. I heard the call of a Raven as he circled overhead. Songs were pounding with each heartbeat, and dizziness overcame me again.

Several days later I woke up in a hospital. Evidently I had been in a coma, pronounced dead, and a sheet placed over my body. Then somehow miraculously I was resurrected, rushed to the hospital for observation and treatment, and got well again. Despite all the confusion and chaos, I clearly remember the experience and the songs. Since then, the Raven has always been with me, no matter where I go, from California to Alaska, Washington to New York. Whenever I do ceremonies or healing, he always comes in. I have learned a lot from that Raven. He has protected my life many times when I was traveling. And he has taught me how to use his power to bring others back from death or from a coma. I am still learning secrets from him.

As a teenager I had yet another experience with the reality of death, dreaming, and dying. During summer vacation I had a job as a recreation leader at Chesapeake Beach Amusement Park, Maryland. Back in the 1960s "the beach" was a wild place because gambling casinos were legal. Drugs, alcohol, and crime were rampant, and the beach became a stomping ground for city gangs that frequently poured in from Washington, D.C., Baltimore, Philadelphia, and New York. It also became a summer residence for Indian families seeking work.

I got off work around eleven one night and started the two-mile walk to our beach house on the bay. It was a strange, unusually quiet night. Every so often the silence would be broken by the sad hooting of an owl, and it made cold chills run up my spine. I heard more owls and remembered that their hooting is always a bad sign. I was glad when my partners pulled up and asked me to go partying.

There were ten of us crammed into an old Chevy. We headed down the country road leading to the city. My friends were already pretty drunk, and they handed me the fifth of Old Crow. We were speeding about seventy miles per hour when unexpectedly a large white dog jumped in front of the car. Frank, my Tuscorora friend, stomped on the brakes. We skidded and slammed into a telephone pole. Everyone was thrown out of the vehicle except me.

Blood was everywhere. I remember the screams, the huge bang of crushing metal, a bright red flash of light, and a dead, silent world of darkness. It wasn't until the tow truck came and pulled the car off the telephone pole that they found my pulverized body.

The Iroquois guardian spirit was standing in the field next to the wreckage. He beckoned me to come over to him. To my amazement, I was aware of my soul hovering over the limp, bloody body of a person I once thought was myself.

I remember following the ambulance all the way to the hospital. I watched them bring my body into the emergency room. Doctors and nurses were rushing around. Then it got very quiet as someone said, "It's too late, he's quit breathing." As they pulled the sheet up over my head, I kept trying to tell them I wasn't dead. I couldn't understand why they didn't hear me.

The next instant I was traveling through an abyss of darkness. Far off in the distance I could see a light; it looked like the evening star. It got closer and brighter. Then I found myself standing on the banks of a river, near an Indian village surrounded by thick woods and mountains. The old grandfather spirit was there with me, the same spirit who had been with me when I first died as a child and when I drowned. We got into a canoe, and a party that looked like Mohawk warriors paddled us toward a village of birchbark long houses across the river. I could see a ceremony and many beautiful people dancing in full regalia.

We pulled onto the riverbank and I started to get out, but a sachem put up his hand to hold me back. Behind him a group of Elders came up to greet me. A clan mother edged forward and spoke: "We are your people, spirits of the Earth, and this is the home of your grandmothers. It is not the right time for you to come here to this world; you must go back. The Creator has chosen a special life for you to follow, and you are still young. But in time, you will go far away from your people here to help others and in time you will be forgotten. Here, drink this sacred water, and you will live a long time. Don't be sad, for someday you will see us again. Someday you will know how to use this water to help others in need."

The Elders gave me gifts, special power objects and regalia they said I would use someday in healing and ceremonies. I was led back to the canoe and paddled downriver into a fog. As the fog cleared I discovered that I was under an oxygen tent and in severe pain except for my legs, which had no feeling. Tubes were up my nose, in my mouth, in my arms, and I even had a catheter. I passed out after seeing this horrible sight. I had a broken back, broken pelvic bones, fractured neck, broken ribs, and internal hemorrhaging from damaged kidneys, liver, and spleen. Later I found out that again I had been pronounced clinically dead, but somehow had come back to life, this time as the orderly was pushing my body down to the morgue. I had spent four days in the intensive care unit and another six days in a coma.

When I finally woke up in the hospital room, I was strapped to my bed. I couldn't move anything. I still didn't have any feelings in my legs. Dr. Bohlman, a bone specialist, was sitting next to my bed in consultation with my distraught mother.

"Well, young man," he said, "you've had a pretty rough time, but it looks like you will make it after all. I was going to put a cast on you from head to toe, but didn't want to take a chance by shifting that spine again. That is why we have you strapped in so tightly; we don't want you to move anything."

He paused for a few minutes as if studying my condition. Then he ran a pen up and down my feet, and asked me if I could feel it. There wasn't any kind of sensation: no pain, no tickle and no movement. He shook his head sadly and said, "I'm sorry to tell you this, but I have to be honest. Your spine is seriously damaged, and as a result paralysis has set in. I don't think you will ever walk again."

The impact of his statement made me vomit all over the bed. The nurse cleaned me up and gave me a sedative. In a few moments I was sound asleep. I don't remember how long I lay in that bed like a vegetable, drugged, but it gave me plenty of time to reflect on the death experience. Thinking about my situation made me wish I had stayed dead.

During the recuperation period, I had an extraordinary dream:

I was standing on a very high mountain ridge, bewildered, and wondering how I got there. Even in the dream I knew I was paralyzed and thought about my predicament. There was something strange about the mountains; it was as if I knew I had been there before, and I felt as though I actually belonged where I was standing. An old trail meandered up toward a huge, golden rock somewhat resembling a chimney.

That majestic, golden rock was very enticing and mysterious; it was magnetic. I tried to walk toward it, but I couldn't move; I was still paralyzed. My predicament was so frustrating that I cried in pain. Suddenly, I heard the deep threatening growl of a grizzly bear. She rose up on her haunches, extended her massive arms and sharp claws, and roared in anger. Her long white teeth flashed just above my face as she was about to devour me. I ran with all my might and kept running.

The high mountain trail was rugged and windy; hence I stumbled, fell, and almost got caught by the raging monster whose hot breath was constantly on my backside. I ran harder and faster in an effort to put some distance between us. Just when I thought I was getting ahead, a large gap appeared in the trail. The empty span between where I stood and the other side was formidable. Below me was a three hundred foot drop into a rocky gorge. Behind me was a rapidly approaching, rapacious grizzly bear. At that point, I was confronted with four precarious choices: turn around and fight without a weapon; somehow manage to sidestep her onslaught and run back to where I had started; commit suicide by jumping into the gorge; or back up a few yards, arouse the last bit of strength left in my aching body, and attempt to leap to the other side. I decided to jump to the other side, and barely made it. Shaking, I pulled myself up. The grizzly bear was standing on the other side of the cliff, still growling, swaying back and forth. Her two big yellow eyes were piercing. It was as if she were saying, "We are not finished yet, and I will see you again."

When I was younger I really didn't understand what these experiences meant. Death and dying, healing and being granted an opportunity to live again can be terrifying to a young person not prepared for such traumatic experiences. But I realize now that this is the school of shamanhood. It is through such experiences, if one truly lives through it, that one becomes a Native healer. In this kind of school we learn about fear, anger, hate, confusion. We learn about other worlds and how to travel between both. We learn about our strengths and weaknesses, power, love, reality, healing, and life itself. We learn that there are, indeed, two separate but interrelated worlds of existence, the physical and the spiritual. The door between these two worlds is via dreams.

It is through dreams that we get our calling. It is through dreams and later visions that we discover our guardian spirit. It is through dreams that we learn it is perfectly natural to call upon supernatural aid when all other resources fail us, that nobody can make it alone. It is through dreams that we get our spiritual knowledge, power objects, doctor tools, and acquire certain forms of knowledge to become Native healers.

3 ▼ POWER DREAMS

▼   ▼   ▼   ▼   ▼   ▼

POWER COMES IN DREAMS. I AM NOT TALKING ABOUT ORDI-
nary dreams in which the subconscious mind works
on what we have absorbed during daily life, the kind
we can't remember because the dreams are not important. I am not talking about fantasies or even creative imagination.

I am, however, talking about a part of the mind-
brain complex that allows us to see realities beyond
the physical world; or to see the physical world while
we are sound asleep. I am not talking about the kinds
of dreams our own mind creates, but dreams we get
from spirits. Both kinds are, indeed, real because the
Indians know that the dream world is the real world.

It exists in what psychologists like Carl Jung (1933) have called the unconscious part of the mind-brain complex. (And it should be mentioned that Jung learned this knowledge from medicine men, though this is not generally known. See *Modern Man in Search of a Soul and Dreams, Memories, Reflections.*)

According to modern psychologists there are two parts to the brain and mind. (According to shamanistic knowledge there are three parts, the last being the spinal column and seat of the spirit.) This is known as "split-brain theory." The conscious mind is directly connected to the left side of the brain. It is influenced by the five senses, and it is the basis for the rational, logical, linear, and digital way of thinking. It is considered the new mind-brain complex and is masculine oriented; it dominates the modern Western way of thinking.

The right side of your brain is directly connected to, and influenced by, the unconscious part of the mind. It is considered the old brain; hence it is primitive and feminine oriented. It is influenced by ancient and natural symbols, creative imagination, instinct, and intuition. It is the spiritual way of thinking. The unconscious part of our mind-brain complex is also the seat of powers of clairvoyance, ESP, telekinesis, clairaudience, precognition, soul-travel, dreams, and visions.

In shamanic training we are taught to develop a holistic way of perceiving and thinking, to use both hemispheres of the mind-brain complex. However, the basis of shamanic thinking and training first starts in the right hemisphere, the old-brain unconscious side of the mind where dreams originate. Dreams can be created by the unconscious mind itself or by spirits that are outside of our minds. We consider spirits per se to be real entities and a source of power. They live around us in the physical world, in the spiritual world, and in outer space. It is difficult for them to communicate with us while we are awake because the conscious mind tries to dominate our thinking patterns; it suppresses all subconscious content and tries to rationalize any reality that does not fit its physical and sensual pattern of verification. Thus, as part of the shamanistic training we are taught how to make the appropriate psychic switch from the conscious to the unconscious, from the logical to the intuitive, from the physical to the spiritual; and we learn that unconscious forms of reality and knowledge are natural sources of human mental power.

Most people in Western society (including non-traditional Natives) primarily think on the conscious level. They have not been taught about the other parts of the mind-brain complex, and most of them have never experienced that there is more to reality than the physical dimension. But dreams, spirits, unconscious archaic symbols, and intuitive/psychic forms of reality and knowledge do not compute with the logical intellect. Hence when average persons encounter something "psychic" or mystical in a dream, for example a talking animal, bird, ghost, or guardian spirit, their minds do not know how to handle or process it. The "phenomena," as they call it, are something beyond their normal grasp. They have spent most of their lives stimulating, developing, and using the conscious mind; hence the subconscious mind is forbidden territory. It does not exist for them. To ignore it, they believe, is the best way to deal with it.

A medicine man or woman must start from the right-brain, subconscious part of the mind. That is where nature has programmed the Indian to think. That is where the ancient genetic knowledge is stored, both physically in the old-brain and psychically in the old-mind system. Thus dreams become one of the first learning tools for Native healers to use in order to develop their innate and spiritual powers, which, by the way, are fully human.

The conscious mind-brain is limited by the physical world and its realities; the subconscious mind is infinite. It is limited only by a person's degree of power, training, development, and courage. But it can also be limited by spiritual guardians and territorial entities and by fear of the unknown. Perhaps for this reason the subconscious is considered a separate universe rarely explored except by a medicine man or woman. Hence to become a medicine person you must also become an explorer, and adventurer, a warrior, and a leader. You must have that something special that drives you into new frontiers with the commitment and understanding that you might never come back. Dreams are therefore dangerous.

To become a medicine man or woman you must learn to be a lonely person because human beings won't really understand you. People don't know how to relate to a "dreamer." You do not fit their norm, their reality. To the average Westerner (and some Indians for that matter) Native healers are considered weird, perhaps because they have weird dreams, dreams about dead people, spirit beings, talking animals and birds, singing rocks, monsters, outer space people, and other worlds. Such has been the case with me.

Before I could become a Native healer, I had to learn how to develop my dreams. As a young child I had nightmares, encounters with monsters, premonitions of accidents or illnesses, disasters that came true, changes in the weather before they occurred, discussions with talking animals, birds, fish, snakes, and dead relatives, and even trips to other planets in flying saucers. I had dreams of falling off cliffs, drowning, being chased by people who tried to kill me, monsters that tried to rip me apart, sleeping in a nest full of snakes, flying over cities, attending parties and gatherings, meeting people who in later years became a friend or spouse, and even dreams about my children before they were born. I actually "saw" my children before they became a physical reality.

My family and friends were scared of me because I would tell them about bad dreams that came true. People don't want to hear premonitions of an illness or forewarning of an accident. But they liked the good dreams, such as the time I told my uncle what horse to bet on two days before he went to the races and won!

We are taught in the Indian way that dreams are sacred. When people have dreams they don't understand, they are taught to seek counsel from an Elder or a medicine man or woman. We are taught to take tobacco, a gift, or money donation and ask the wise one to interpret our dreams for us. This is how I met medicine people from different tribes. Eventually these people started to take a special interest in me. They began to teach me how to remember and study my dreams. They taught me how to distinguish the difference between a dream that is ordinary and a dream that was a definite message or communication. They taught me how to use creative imagination to make the dreams more clear, to remember certain dreams, to cultivate dream power in order to "see" in a clairvoyant way. They even taught me how to change dreams to prevent an accident or injury, or to communicate long distance with others in a dream. They taught me how to acquire a dream ally and how to learn from the animals, birds, ghosts, spirits who taught me secrets of herbs, medicine-making, and healing in dreams. And because of some of my dreams, they said I was chosen to become a Native healer and spiritual teacher—or what people call a medicine man.

We can share some dreams with other people, but some dreams we must keep to ourselves. If we share a "power dream" with the wrong person, we can get sick or lose the power. Power dreams that give us pain must be doctored by a Native healer. We hire him or her to take the pain out, or to teach us how to overcome the pain and use it as an ally. I have had a number of dreams involving pain. Some were good and some were bad. For example, I once had a dream that an elderly Indian man kept trying to stab me in the stomach with a fishing harpoon. I got very sick afterward and developed ulcers and stomach pain. I went to one of my elderly medicine mentors with to- bacco, Indian blankets, a $100 bill, and some salmon. I forgot to tell him about the dream when I asked him to doctor me. All I could think about at the time was the pain and the diagnosis by the White doctor (physician). The elderly Native healer started praying, singing, and dancing for me that night. During the middle of the healing session he stopped and said, "My spirits told me you had a bad dream about an elderly man from the coast who kept trying to stab you with a fishing harpoon. Is this true?" In amaze- ment, I said, "Yes. I forgot all about that dream." He scolded me for not paying attention to my dream. He said I was being shown an act of sorcery against my life, and I should have heeded the warning, and "seen" what was going on and defended myself against it. Since I did not, I became sick. However, I learned through that mistake. The healer taught me that I should immediately stop such a dream. He gave me an analogy: "Your dreams are like a movie. It has different pictures that go in such rapid succession that all you see is the whole picture moving. You can train your mind and brain either to slow the process down or to stop it at any particular point; then you can take something out. Next time try to focus on the dream, slow it down, and then freeze it. Remove the weapon from the attacker and destroy it. Another technique is to call in your dream ally such as the bear as a protector and have him defend you."

I didn't fully understand and sought further clarification. He continued: "Remember when you were a little child and you had bad dreams about monsters, snakes, etc.?" I said, "Yes." "Well, what did you do? At first you ran from the dreams, lived in nightmares and torment. Then after a while you got tired of it and decided to fight it yourself. Remember, you stood up to the monster in your dreams. You tried to fight it, but it was too big and powerful. So you cried out for help. And who came in to help you? Sometimes it was the bear, sometimes a wolf, sometimes a warrior, or a wise old man. These are your dream allies, advisers, and protectors. We all have them. You just need to learn how to use them again, how to keep them alive and active through creative dream training, meditation, and vision seeking in the sweat lodge. The more you practice, the better you will become. Hawks and eagles eat snakes, snakes eat other snakes, water puts out fire, certain spirits catch shadows, warriors fight other warriors, some animals are stronger than other animals, some fish eat other fish. Use these in your dreams. Visualizing a ring of fire can protect you against enemies or demons. You can even create a fog around you or make yourself invisible so that the other person or thing can't find you. Understand?"

The elderly medicine man took the bad dream

away by his knowledge and power and he also took the pain out of my body by removing the harpoon. Such things do not show up on the X-ray machine and are not visible to the naked eye, but they are apparent to the spiritual eye. Thus dreams in this context move into the realm of clairvoyance.

Some medicine people have difficulty in developing their dreams. Even shamans can have trouble becoming dreamers during their apprenticeship and sometimes during their professional life. Different tribes handle the situation with different techniques. Some of the medicine people in the southwest use datura medicine, or what is called jimson weed. It is a narcotic herb and can be very dangerous if not handled in the right and proper way and used under strict supervision. Stanley Smart, an elderly friend of mine who is a well-known medicine man in Nevada, uses peyote. That is his main medicine because he is what our Native people call a Road Man. I have never used datura, but I did try peyote once with Stanley during one of his sacred ceremonies. I didn't like it at all. I got terrible headaches and was nauseated; my heart bothered me for three days, and my vision was completely distorted. If I had any dreams I didn't remember them. I found out later that peyote has natural arsenic poison in it. And it really tastes gross!

My mentors taught me a different way. Most of my training in dreaming was through practicing meditation in the sweat lodge. Occasionally I had to use the power of mugwort, a non-narcotic herb, during the full moon, but the full development came through

vision-seeking at specific power centers. The meditation I was taught is a combination of ritual and self-
hypnosis. During the earlier stages I had to sit by a
sacred fire, pray, and stare into it for hours, days, and
nights. All this time I fasted: no food, no water, no
sex, no socializing. All I could drink was a soupy form
of acorn meal mush. I had to stay in an isolated spot
in the woods and concentrate on how to get into my
subconscious mind. A series of prayer formulas, singing, and chanting aided me in the process. I also had
to discipline myself to remember my dreams, but I
was not allowed to use a notebook and pencil or tape
recorder. There were times when I could not remember specific dreams. The elderly medicine man then
showed me how to gather the sacred mugwort herb
during the full moon, talk to it and ask for help, then
boil it and drink the tea. I was also taught how to
make special prayers to Grandmother Moon in order
to learn how to use the lunar light and power to open
up the faculties of my mind. The warm leaves from
the plant were placed in a headband and wrapped
lightly around my skull. The herbs help absorb the
power of the Moon and transfer it into the brain cells
and mind energy field. I had to pray something like
this:

> *Grandmother Moon, I come before you in a
> humble manner and ask for your help. The Great
> Creator put you here on this Earth from the very
> Beginning of Time. You have a special power and
> purpose. I offer you this tobacco as payment and I*

ask that you shine your light and power into my herbal tea and the wormwood leaves. With the use of these two powers I ask that you open up my spiritual mind so I can see my dreams clearly and remember my dreams. I ask that you talk to me in a dream, language, and vision that I can understand and show me how to become a dreamer.

I did this for four nights during the full moon and drank one cup of tea per night. (Man is it bitter!) The whole time I sat by the sacred fire focusing my attention on the color, sound, and movement of the flames as they danced within the fire. I was taught to relax and breathe, inhale deeply, count to four, then exhale very slowly, counting backward from seven. This process was repeated four times throughout the night after drinking the tea. It worked for me.

The other herb that helped me was the wild Native tobacco. You can hardly find it anymore since the Forest Service and timber companies wiped it out. But it is strong medicine for dreaming, very different from domesticated tobacco. Wild tobacco has a real kick to it in terms of taste and power, and it can help put you in a hypnogogic state.

Smoking and praying with tobacco is the main ingredient for almost all Native ceremonies; it is probably the most ancient ritual we have, and it is still being used today. The tobacco is offered to the spirits as payment in exchange for their assistance. Smoke from tobacco offered to the Great Spirit of the Universe, our Creator, carries our prayers to him from the physical world into the spirit world. The smoky color, movement, silence, and rhythm represent the spirits of our ancestors. When they first appear they take on a similar smoky form.

Sometimes dreams first come as if behind a screen of smoke, and a person in training must learn how to focus on that smoke, follow it into the spirit world, and clear it away so that the vision will manifest. All this takes time, training, and discipline in privacy and in a quiet environment. I suppose it is a way of programming the mind, because once the training is completed you can slip into that state of mind any time and any place.

In later stages of dreaming I was taught how to see myself or other people or places in my dreams. I would pre-envision the scene, pre-enact a particular scene, then pre-attain it. The same process, or what we call "medicine making," is used for deer hunting when the hunter prepares for the hunt in the sacred sweat lodge, or when the gambler prepares for the Indian sport called handgame. Olympic athletes are now taught a similar mental process called "autogenic training."

Of all the methods for dream training, however, I believe the sacred sweat lodge is the most powerful. When we go into the sweat lodge we are going into the womb of our Mother Earth. We are naked, hence stripped of ego, self-importance, and whatever credentials a person may be accustomed to flashing in life. We enter the sacred sweat lodge on all fours like the bear and our animal relations, or like the turtle so close to the electromagnetic force field of the earth. We go from the light into the darkness, from the known into the unknown, from the physical world into the spiritual world, from the conscious into the unconscious. The fasting, sweating, purification, and total relaxation put us into an altered state of consciousness. Here we can transcend all humanness and become more spirit-like.

The small entrance to the sweat lodge can serve as a symbolic doorway, a key to unlocking hidden mysteries and secrets within the vast universe of our subconscious mind. Sometimes we need a special kind of key or technique to get into the dream world. The ancient archetypes and symbols laying dormant in our unconscious mind become activated while meditating in the sweat lodge. The privacy and isolation offer a special environment for the neophyte to use as a means to analyze and decipher the most complex dreams. It is a perfect place to practice dreaming. We can use the sweat lodge as a supernatural aid and psychological tool to transform dreams into visions. I have had some of my strongest visions in the sweat lodge.

The voices of our ancestors talk to us in the sweat lodge. That is the way it has always been. The spirits feel more comfortable visiting us in a sacred and spiritual environment. It is easier to discover a dream ally while dreaming in the sweat lodge. Our power allies from Nature and the spirit world can communicate to us easier because our mind is not being bombarded with radio music, television movies, advertisements, human chatter, and noise pollution. As an example, a number of years ago we were conducting a purification sweat, which is held to cleanse our mind, body, and soul. We had been in the sweat lodge for a long time when several of us thought that we heard the cry of an eagle in there. Some of the men left, and the remaining few decided to sleep in the sweat lodge through the night. We all had dreams about eagles. We compared our dreams in the morning and discovered that each one had been given a special personal message. I had a dream that I was high up on a mountain top seeking a vision and an eagle flew down to visit with me. He said: "Do you want to learn how to fly? Would you like to be able to see long distance like I can? I will share my power with you in doctoring. Just get on for a ride." So in the dream I saw myself climbing on the back of a giant eagle. We flew over valleys, fields, farms, and mountains; higher and higher we went into the sky. I was so happy and relaxed, and it was an extremely peaceful experience. I had a feeling of freedom that is difficult to explain. Ever since I have used that dream as a form of stress management and for doctoring other people. Whenever I feel uptight and under a lot of stress, I simply close my eyes for a few moments, do my breathing exercises, go into a hypnogogic state, and relive the dream. Sometimes I can even see myself turning into the eagle flying through the sky, and I can feel the wind blowing through my feathers. A few moments of this kind of meditation and all the stress is gone. I am totally relaxed.

A few months after I had that dream in the sweat lodge, I went on a vision quest. What I saw in the dream became a reality, except for the actual physical part of climbing on the eagle's back and going for a ride. That part came in spiritual form, as a vision, only this time the eagle told me secrets about healing and spirituality that I cannot share. A few days later while hunting I found a golden eagle near a sacred mountain. So the dream ally became a power ally, which in turn manifested physically and became doctoring and ceremonial regalia. The dream became a vision, the vision became another form of reality and a means to acquire power. That kind of power is needed in order to become a medicine man or woman and serve the people.

I have mentioned that we are chosen to become Native healers through dreams. An ancestor, ghost, animal, spirit, force, power, or the Great Creator talks to us in dreams. They tell us that we have been chosen to be a certain kind of medicine person, and they give specific instructions on how to use their medicine and power. In most cases the dream ally or guardian spirit also gives us a song, and it is sacred and special. It can be a dreaming song, seeing song, love song, hunting song, fishing song, protection song, traveling song, healing song. Sometimes they teach us several songs, each for a different purpose. When we sing the songs they teach, we are calling in their power for assistance, the power of Bear, Eagle, Raven, Hummingbird, Dolphin, Coyote, Wolf, King Snake, Buffalo, Elk, Beaver, Turtle, Rock People, or even a sacred mountain, waterfall, underground spirit, or lightning and thunder. Sometimes one spirit helps us, sometimes many different spirits.

We need help and guidance when these things first start coming in dreams. At first the dream may not be clear, or we may not be developed enough to hear and understand what the dream ally or power is trying to communicate. That is why we go to a medicine man or woman for counseling. We approach them with respect, with tobacco, a gift, and usually a money donation. We talk to them confidentially about the dream and ask for interpretation. Such dreams do not always mean that someone will become a medicine person. But if you are meant to be a shaman you receive your calling, initiation into shamanhood, and acquire your power through dreams.

Perhaps the most difficult thing about dreams is believing in them. At first when you hear dream allies or spirits talking to you, you might think it is your imagination going crazy. Your conscious, rational mind will do everything to block it out, so you must be persistent. To become a medicine man or woman, you must have faith in the Great Creator, the dreams, the spirits, the good powers, and in yourself. At first dreams bring the calling and initiation into shamanhood; later they become tools for self-discovery, spiritual self-development, protection, diagnosis, and healing. After the dream comes the vision quest, and after the vision quest the apprenticeship under an older medicine man or woman. I have had dreams about my mentors years before I met them. Dreams guide our development and keep us on the shamanistic path. But there is a difference between dreams and visions.

4 ▼ VISION SEEKING AND
POWER QUESTS

▼   ▼   ▼   ▼   ▼   ▼

WHO ARE WE, AND WHY ARE WE ON THIS EARTH? TO FIND
out, we must seek a vision. Chief Crazy Horse said
around 1850: "A very good vision is needed for life,
and the man who has it must follow it—as the eagle
seeks the deepest blue of the sky."

In order to have a vision we must turn to the Great
Creator, Mother Earth, and our relations in Nature.
We must enter the dream world and the deeper levels
of our own mind, to the ancient archetypal images in
our unconscious, to our very soul. We need a vision in
order to guide us through life, to give meaning to our

life, to give us strength and protection, and to find answers to those mysterious questions and experiences that plague our life with pain and suffering.

It is through the vision quest that we get our power. Through a vision quest we can discover who we really are. There are places in Nature we can visit in the right way and find out directly from the Source of Creation what our own power is, or what kind of power we should have.

With the vision comes supernatural aid, or what you might call a totem or spirit guardian. This spirit ally can become our adviser, teacher, protector, and secret partner. It is through the vision quest that we receive confirmation to be a Native healer and learn what kind of healer we will be. And, as stated earlier, dreams and dreaming are a prerequisite for vision seeking.

Dreams are different from visions. Dreams can be vague and fleeting, sometimes confusing. Sometimes they come in sets like a puzzle; each part must be studied, deciphered, and understood as it relates to the whole series. Dreams can be induced or occur spontaneously. Visions are clear, colorful, dynamic, and longer lasting. A person can forget a dream but never a vision. Dreams are the doorway to the spirit world; the vision is the spirit world.

There is a difference between a vision quest and a power quest. A vision quest is to seek a vision. Visions are used to advise us and to guide our lives, to tell, show, and teach us things about ourselves, about life, and about Nature. We seek visions to find solutions to problems, to get a power ally or spirit ally, or to find out who we are, where we came from, what our purpose and function in life is.

I have been on many vision quests for many different reasons. Sometimes I have sought visions from the spirit world on how to heal a person with an incurable disease, or someone who was troubled or lost in life, had marital problems, or had problems on the job. Those kinds of visions, either in the sweat house or different places in Nature, we call lamenting.

The power quest is different. The vision quest provides us with the opportunity to find out what kinds of power we as human beings have inside of us. With the power quest we are looking for another kind of power. We go out to a certain place in Nature that is a source of power and was put there in the Beginning. It could be a place where men train to be warriors or women train to be seers, or people quest for gambling power. It could be a place where people go for good luck and wealth. It could be a place in Nature where one goes to train for strength and agility in sports or a place high in the alpine lakes where one goes to train for bravery and courage. There are places in Nature where our Native people train for protection or for long life. You can learn, through myths, legends, and the history of the tribes in a geographical area, what places the local Native people went to and for what reasons. A number of anthropologists (Park, Kroeber, Bean, and Buckley) have documented evidence of this training.

If you want to train for doctor power, you have to

go to a doctor training grounds. But just because you go there and do everything right, it does not mean you will get that power. Sometimes people might want something because they are selfish or their intentions are not good. As a backlash, they might just get what the Great Creator thinks they need rather than what they want. For example, I didn't ask to become a Native healer. I even tried to take the medicine power out by power training. It didn't work. I am still stuck with it, because that is what I am meant to be. I guess the Elders knew this all along, and that is why they kept teaching and training me over the past forty years. I went on a power quest to acquire good luck in gambling and became a Native healer instead!

As you can see, there are many different kinds of power quests and vision quests. Most quests require purification in the sweat lodge as preparation for a mountain or cave quest. Or the quest could be by the ocean, beneath a waterfall, in a forest such as the ancient Redwood forest, on a high butte, in the middle of the desert, or inside the kiva or sweat lodge. For many young girls it is during their first puberty rite, or what we call the moontime ceremony, or the flower dance. So the puberty rite is also a power quest. Even childbirth can be a source of power and a power quest for the woman and child, if they know how to handle it.

The vision quest or power quest depends upon the geographical area you come from and the tribe you are in. Even the White people had the vision quest long ago in European cultures. The Blacks still have it, and some Asians and Hawaiians still use it. Many Native tribes use the vision quest, although some have lost it. You may go on one quest or many, depending on your tribe, your degree of spiritual development, and your destiny.

The quest might be four days and nights, seven days and nights, or ten days and nights, or could be as long as thirty days and nights (one full moon period). I have gone through all the different kinds of power quests during my life-long shamanistic apprenticeship, and I know I have to go on more. Wallace Black Elk, an elderly Lakota medicine man, has gone on forty different vision quests. To me, that is a remarkable commitment and accomplishment for spiritual service.

There have even been times that I have had to go thirty days and nights with no food and no water and hiked every inch of the way in the sacred high country up to the highest mountain. I was not allowed to drive up there in a four-wheel drive. I fasted and was allowed only a small portion of acorn soup daily. There was no cheating along the way. You have to suffer and sacrifice and prove that you are worthy to go to these places. You have to prepare yourself in the right and proper way. If you get a negative attitude about it, don't even try to embark on a power quest.

You ask: "Who am I? Who am I, really, Great Creator, Mother Earth, and all my relations in Nature? Who is the real ME inside? Where did I come from? What is my purpose and function in life? What do you want me to do? What do you want me to be, Great Spirit?"

Sometimes the knowledge and information come through a dream or a vision, or sometimes they manifest directly in front of you like a movie projector shining onto a screen. Sometimes they show up in a symbolic way, in a dream or in your mind, or appear on the side of a mountain or in a cloud. The power and vision can appear through the spirit of the wind or as the appearance of a ghost. They manifest in many ways because we are all different and the places in Nature are all different.

Sometimes when we are just sitting on a vision quest, we enter into what has been called an altered state of consciousness; we switch into a different state, like changing the channels on a television in your head. In your mind you can see everything so clearly, and you are shown visions.

Most Native tribes and traditional people use the sacred sweat lodge as a means to prepare for a vision quest. During this time they are instructed by the Elders to abstain from drugs, alcohol, certain foods, and even sex for approximately four days and nights. The sweat lodge and abstaining are used to purify one's mind, body, and soul. In some tribes, the neophyte is placed in a hot mineral spring or in a waterfall for this purpose. In northwestern California the Native people sometimes purified themselves by "smoke pits" in addition to the sweathouse. They built a fire pit in the ground, waited until the wood became coals, then placed heaps of fresh Douglas fir boughs upon the coals and thoroughly smudged themselves. This method serves to rid one of human scent, which we believe the spirits consider repulsive.

Purification is the first step toward the acquisition of power or toward making contact with a power source, so it must be taken seriously. Purification also requires disciplining one's thoughts and actions—not thinking about favorite foods, abstaining from specific foods and drinks, not thinking about sex, and abstaining from sex during the spiritual training period. We must clear our minds from any interference, internal dialogue, and personal desires, and we must focus specifically on the task at hand. So although our Native people consider sex as natural, beautiful, and special, they keep things in perspective by sacrificing this part of humanness in an attempt to get more into their spiritual side. In order to be successful, you must focus all your attention, energy, and physical strength into the acquisition of power.

There are other types of rules that we apply at this time that deal with understanding how certain kinds of energy work. For example, men must not be around menstruating women and the women's "moontime" energy during this time, or it could hurt them both. Certain types of energies and powers just don't mix properly. By the same token, a woman should not undergo a vision quest or power quest (other than the moontime ceremony) while she is on her menses. The spirits do not want that kind of energy in their power center, as it does not mix properly. The same can be said for social interaction. It is best to avoid eating with people who are on drugs or alcohol or who may be a potential source of negative energy. Thus fasting, isolation, abstaining from sex, and avoiding other people's energies are part of the purification process. It is through purification that we rid ourselves of our own negative energies and attempt to become a vessel for positive, creative energies.

When we go into the sacred sweat lodge we are purifying our mind, body, and soul with the four powers of creation. We call upon the four colors and the four elements to help us; we are in a sense attempting to replicate creation itself in the Beginning. The powers of the air, fire, earth, and water are used to purify our mind, body, soul, and spirit. That is the natural law and method as we understand it. We have to center ourselves with these four elements in order to gather re-creation and strength.

In addition, part of the preparation requires physical exertion. We might have to walk, hike, or run all the way from the sweat lodge to a high butte. We might even have to swim or crawl to the power center after staying in the sweat lodge and fasting for one hour or for one whole day. Once again, the process depends on the kind of power we intend to quest for and where the power center is located. It can be different for each tribe or geographical area.

Suffering and sacrifice are part of the price involved. You take all your normal human actions, all your basic human needs, all your petty hang-ups, all your personal desires, all the things that mean the most to you in life, and you put them temporarily to the side. In this way, you strip yourself down to becoming like an innocent child once again—a cosmic child in the womb of creation.

By getting in contact with your own inner self, you know when power flows through you. When you get a vision, you have earned it, have qualified for it. Nobody can take that away from you. Once you get a vision or power the hard way, you never lose it.

There is anthropological research on many different tribes and the ways they saw visions and how they went for power. The Navajo, Hopi, Iroquois Six Nations, Chippewa, Sioux, Cree, Blackfoot, Crow, Cherokee, Shoshone or Pomo, and Wintun all have their ways. The Native people in Alaska have their way. Eastern Woodland Indians, desert Indians, plains Indians, coastal Indians, river Indians, ocean Indians all have their ways. Native people everywhere had different kinds of vision or power quests, but basically they are all the same because they approached them with respect and with humbleness. And they made basically the same sacrifices. That kind of training is strict and requires discipline.

Let me give you other examples. One time when I was having problems with money and needed help, I went on a power quest. It's not that I wanted to be greedy; it's just that I was having financial hardships like other people. I went to see an old medicine man, not a doctor or healer but more of a ceremonial leader. I took him tobacco, a hundred dollar bill, some nice fish, and some deer meat. I chopped wood for him, then I sat down and explained: "Grandfather, I'm having too much trouble with my life. I have too many bills and too many financial problems. Isn't there some way or somewhere that I can go out in Nature and pray and train? Isn't there a power place in Nature where I can go and break this bad medicine, this bad luck?" He sat there for a long time and said nothing. He just looked around and watched the different birds passing by to check for omens. Then he told me, "Yes."

He then prepared me. There was a power place down along the coast which required five days and nights of questing. (To go to the higher mountains one has to train for ten days and nights.) So for five days and nights I stayed in the sweat house and didn't go into my house. I stayed away from all people. I packed my own firewood. I fasted on acorn soup for five days and nights. I sweated and prayed around the fire. I talked to the Creator and the spirits and the earth and told them about my problem.

On the fifth day, the old medicine man took me to a certain rock along the coast. He had me stay up there all night and talk to the Great Creator, the Mother Earth, the spirits of Nature, and to the spirit of that rock. It was considered a good luck rock, and I asked for good luck. The next morning I had my vision. A woodpecker came in and started pecking on a nearby tree. It wasn't long after that that my prayers were answered and my wishes came true because in a mysterious way I got some money, just enough to pay off my debts. The woodpecker symbolically and spiritually represents wealth.

One time I had a dream that led to a vision quest. I was standing in a field near a small pond at the base of a mountain. I did not recognize the mountain in the dream. I felt so peaceful and happy in that dream place that I wished it would last forever. In the dream I sat down by the little pond wondering if I should jump into it. Then I heard the gentle footsteps of an animal nearby; it was a deer coming through the brush to the water to drink. She stopped and stared at me for a long time, as if to communicate telepathically. But I could not understand what she was trying to say. I knew intuitively that the dream meant something but could not seem to analyze it. I had the same dream three times, so according to Native custom and belief, I went to seek counsel—from a medicine woman who specializes in dream power—and I approached her properly. She told me that I was being guided to a sacred place by the deer. She said I would have to go on a vision quest and try to relive that dream while fasting and praying. The deer would talk to me and tell me secrets.

I did not know where to go, when to go, or what to do, so I asked for further guidance. The elderly medicine woman said that this was a very sacred and special dream. She said I needed the Deer power and medicine in order to put me in balance because I was too "macho," too male thinking. The deer was a feminine power and symbol from my unconscious and the spirit world, and it represented power from the South. So she agreed to help me.

A few months later in summer I prepared for the quest. I had to fast and purify myself in the sacred sweat lodge, hike thirty miles into the Marble Mountains, and set up my altar for a quest. The medicine woman had told me exactly where to go; she said the place in the dream was a dream power site that her people had used for doctor training. And she was right. The old Indian trail led me directly to a spot I had seen in a dream several months earlier.

By the time I got to the power center and set up camp, I was exhausted, hungry, and thirsty. I had been warned not to eat deer meat for at least one month prior to the quest, during the quest, and for one full moon after the quest. So the only supplement I took with me was fresh corn soup; just enough nourishment and moisture to keep me going. I was already into the seventh day of fasting. I made my altar and started a sacred fire, introduced myself to the Great Creator, the spirit of the mountain, and all my relations in Nature. I offered them tobacco, burned a few sacred angelica roots as payment, and asked for permission to be in their territory. The sun hung low. The bird people were singing their evening song, and a few small fish began jumping out of the water after bugs. I have never felt such peace and tranquility. I sat by the fire just taking in all the splendor and beauty of Nature and waited patiently for a vision. I had a deer antler pipe that the medicine woman had given me as a gift to smoke and pray with.

After a few hours I became drowsy, rolled over on the lush meadow grass, and went to sleep. I began to dream of deer—white deer, red deer, yellow deer and black deer. At first four separate deer were coming from each direction. Then I began to see herds of deer everywhere, deer in meadows, deer running through woods, deer grazing in meadows and farm lands. Then I saw deer being hunted in the old way, with proper medicine-making and ceremony. The dream became horrible as I saw White men and Indians hunting when they were drunk, unclean, and just out for the sport. I saw deer slaughtered in every conceivable way, wasted for their antlers or choice chunks of meat. I saw whole herds crying as they were massacred. I saw fawns mangled by passing cars on the highways and left to die, twisted in pain. I began crying in my sleep. I tried to wake up from the dream but couldn't. Then the dream began to change as I heard singing.

The songs led me to my wife's people dancing and singing in their most sacred ceremony, the White Deerskin Dance. I saw myself dancing in this ceremony for what seemed like ages, while in the background I could hear the ceremonial leader repeating the ancient story about how the world was first created with the help of the Deer People. The sacred White Deerskin Dance is a re-enactment of the original creation.

My dream was suddenly interrupted by the sound

of someone walking close by, in a circular pattern. I jumped up from a deep sleep. After carefully scrutinizing the surroundings, I decided it was just my imagination or else a small animal. I sat up and began praying again.

A couple of hours later I went back to sleep and dreamed again. I was standing in a meadow watching a strong, handsome, proud buck come down a mountain trail. He walked up to me and began talking: "I am glad that you have come to visit us. I have a message I want to share with you. Try to remember it and share it with your people.

"We Deer are sacred beings. We were put here on the Earth for a reason and purpose. Take a good look at my body, you see how healthy I am. I know exactly what plants and herbs to eat to be healthy and strong. So when you humans eat our flesh you are getting all the vitamins, minerals, proteins, and nourishment you need to be strong and healthy. You see how I live. I can run up and down mountains, swim rivers, and travel long distances. When you eat my flesh you become strong with endurance like me.

"I also know how to doctor myself when I get sick or wounded. After a forest fire I lie down in the coals and smoke myself. In this way I get rid of all the ticks and fleas. When the burn has cooled I chew the charcoals to flush the parasites and worms out of my body. When I become wounded from a fight or accident I know exactly what herbs to eat, and how to pack the medicine mud into my wounds; if need be, I will even go down to the ocean and bathe in the salt water or in mineral springs.

"You see my eyes and ears. I can see long distances and hear long distances. So when you eat my flesh you are getting medicine and natural power for long life; to be able to have good hearing and eyesight.

"Everything you humans need to live and survive can come from my people. My body can sustain a whole human family for a long period of time. There is just enough hide to make you a shirt, a dress, and moccasins. There is just enough brains to tan the hide, and the string for sewing can come from my backstrap and hind legs. I even have a needle for you near my hoofs. The hoofs can be used as rattles to sing sacred songs. There are other powers we can share with those who are deserving; as in assistance during childbirth for a woman in labor.

"Now I ask, why do your people no longer respect me? We are a sacred people, not just a food source. We have been placed here on the earth, by the Great Creator to help you. Why do you no longer follow the custom and laws we agreed upon? We are willing to give you humans all these gifts. In exchange we ask only that you treat us with respect. You must be clean when you hunt us, make your medicine in the sweat lodge, offer tobacco and prayer as agreed upon in the Beginning. Women on the menses or bleeding during childbirth are not allowed to touch, cook, or handle our meat or medicine. The woman's power and negative discharge at that time can hurt us; certain powers in this world just don't mix. Any man who hunts us while unclean and with disrespect will be punished. If you hurt us we will hurt you. That has always been the agreement between us. All tribes of your people across the land know this law. This law may be ancient but it is not archaic; it is eternal. White people and other races are subject to the same law. For every action there is a reaction. Thus humans who do not respect the laws will be penalized; accidents, sickness, disease, arthritis, heart attacks, insanity, and even death may occur to the violators. The White man's doctor will not know how to cure such sicknesses caused by transgression, so teach your people to respect the old ways and to show respect to us."

Once again I awoke from the deep sleep by the sound of someone walking around me in a circle. The steps were heavy enough to be human but light in motion, the way a woman walks. I thought to myself, this is strange. What would a woman be doing up here late at night, all by herself? Then my conscious mind began to rationalize: I told myself it was probably one of those college students conducting research. I thought: I don't need people around me at a time like this to ruin the vision quest. Man, I hope it isn't a woman, especially one who is on her menses, because that could break my medicine. And if she is good looking, it could break my power of concentration. I've got to keep clean thoughts.

I jumped up once again, and looked around. I could hear the footsteps and tried to judge the weight and size of the person making the noise. I totally ruled out the possibility of a man, unless he was very slight in build. It had to be a woman. Just my luck, I thought. Another test to go through! Then I hollered at her, "Hey," I said, "I know you are out there. Who are you, what do you want?" The walking continued, but there was no response. So I put more wood on the fire to create more light. I got up, looked around in the bushes that were highlighted by the fire, and I even went into the shadows. I found nothing. So I thought I would scare the person out, and hollered: "Hey, whoever is hiding out there! I have a gun. I am going to start shooting unless you come out and talk to me!" (I didn't really have a gun.) Still no response. So I figured it was just my imagination playing tricks on me; after all, I was starved and exhausted. That, with the high altitude, could cause hallucination.

For the fourth time I went back to sleep. This time I did not dream, but I was disturbed by the incident and could not sleep well. My mind began to wander, and I thought about stories I had heard about crazy people on drugs, hiding in the woods. There had been accounts of such city people killing backpackers or forest rangers. Then I thought, This must be a test of my faith in the power. I will have to rely on the power to protect me.

I was just about asleep when the walking started again. This time I decided to lie still and see how close it would come. Whoever or whatever it was walked around me four times and stopped. Then dead silence. I sat so still I even held my breath and waited for it to come closer. Then I felt hot breath on my ear. Terrified, I jumped up in defense. To my amazement, there was a young doe standing directly in front of me, the same deer I had seen in my dream several months ago. As if by magic, I watched her turn into a beautiful young Native woman with long black hair that was braided and wrapped in otter fur. She wore a maple bark dress with red flicker feathers dangling from the sides, and her huge eyes were almond shaped like a deer. She said: "I am the Deer spirit who talked to you in a dream. I am happy that you finally came to visit me in my home. I have been waiting to give you a gift. You will never be a good hunter, but when the time comes, if you need food I will tell you what to do. My medicine is for healing, not for hunting. This is my song and this is how you can use my power."

I can't tell you everything the deer spirit told me or I will lose that power and gift. This lengthy account is to demonstrate how significant dreams are, and how dreams help make one a medicine man or woman.

The power and gift a healer gets from a dream must be used to help the people. I use the secrets that deer spoke into my ear to help men who have bad luck in hunting. I also use the power of the deer to interpret dreams for others on certain occasions. Sometimes the deer will appear as a messenger when I am traveling down the highway, becoming my eyes and ears, often warning of danger in the road. But most of all I have used the power of the deer to help balance me in order to qualify for other powers. The deer has taught me patience, gentleness, understanding, love, caring, and the gift of sensitivity in counseling women. The greatest gift she loaned me, however, was the gift of healing.

5 ▼ THE CALLING

▼   ▼   ▼   ▼   ▼   ▼

Anyone who is meant to be a medicine man or woman will know it sooner or later. He or she will be shown in dreams, instructed in dreams, then guided to an older medicine person who will intuitively "know"; and that person will become a mentor. It is as if it has already been arranged somewhere, probably in the dream or spirit world.

Such was the case with me. I went to California during the start of the Red Power movement from the East Coast. I traveled from reservation to reservation during the resurgence era of Indian identity and return to Nativism. I went from Kinzua Dam to Alcatraz Island, to the Pitt River, to Frank's Landing Fishing War, to save the ancient redwoods, and eventually with the G-O Road, Sacred High Country conflict in northwestern California. Sometimes I was with the White Roots of Peace and sometimes with different medicine men such as Mad Bear Anderson, John Fire Lamedeer, Grandpa David Mononge, Thomas Banyaca, Rose Williams, Rolling Thunder, Calvin Rube, Semu, Uncle Billy Mesa, Bonita Matsen, Raymond Legu, Willard Rhoades, Flora Jones, Chief Ed Chilogiun, Martin High Bear, and many more. Indian people were waking up all over this country, traveling from reservation to urban centers, teaching about sacred ways and "return to the blanket." A revitalization of Native religion, beliefs, and practices spread like a flood, and many of us were swept up in the current. We had sacred tobacco burning ceremonies, sweat lodge ceremonies, doctoring ceremonies, moontime rituals, naming rituals, vision quests, potlatches, story-telling sessions, talking circles, and spiritual training. It was a time of intertribal and cross-cultural teaching and learning. For me it became a calling into the medicine ways and an initiation into shamanhood.

During this time I had some of my most powerful dreams—about mountains, forests, old Indian trails, waterfalls, rivers, caves, cliffs, and rock drawings I didn't even know existed. I had dreams about ghosts and spirits I discovered later were elderly medicine men and women, long deceased; dreams about talking animals, birds, fishes, snakes, plants and herbs, old Indian villages, ceremonies, rituals, and even UFO's.

The more I participated in sacred ceremonies and sweats, the more I dreamed. Each dream was a spiritual puzzle and teaching. Little did I realize at the time that these dreams were leading me into a whole new world that exists beyond the physical reality of everyday life. Each one led me to a different elderly medicine person who interpreted my dreams, counseled me in my spiritual growth and development, and put me under apprenticeship to become a Native healer and spiritual teacher for the people. One particular dream, actually a vision, took seven years and over 30,000 miles of traveling to put together. Eventually I had to go on a vision quest to relive each part of it, decipher it, experience it, and fully understand it. In other words, I had to go directly to the vision to get the final power and meaning. It was my movement on the great circle of the medicine wheel, but I cannot share it with others.

A person does not choose his or her mentor; when the student is ready the teacher will come. If you are meant to be trained under the tutelage of a certain elderly mentor, he or she will pick you out of a crowd of thousands. I know, because it has happened to me several times. On a number of occasions I had different medicine people walk up to me and say: "I had a dream about you; you are the young man I have been waiting for. I am meant to be your teacher. When you think you are ready, come and visit me. We will talk about your mysterious dreams and mystical experiences. We will talk to the Great Creator and the good spirits about your destiny; and if it is meant to be, I will make you my apprentice."

Sometimes neophytes will get very sick from strange dreams. That sickness guides them to a certain kind of healer for doctoring. It is through the bad dream, sickness, and pain that the elderly medicine person learns about the neophyte's power.

Not all medicine people are good. Some of them tried to steal my power or were jealous and tried to take away my power while doctoring me. They knew that I was chosen to be a Native healer and ceremonial leader someday, and they tried to stop the process. But these kinds of people, sorcerers or "Indian devils" as we call them, are important in our growth and development. We learn from bad experiences and encounters with evil power. We learn how to defend, protect, and heal ourselves and others who may have had similar experiences but did not have the knowledge or power to pull out of it. We learn by studying the behavior of model figures, good and bad. And we learn from our own stupidity and mistakes.

Over the years I kept having tormenting dreams about grizzly bears. The dream challenger was always stalking me and trying to attack me, and it seemed as though he was trying to devour me. The dreams were always more vivid during or after a sacred sweat lodge ceremony. I went to a number of medicine people for doctoring because of the nightmares. Some helped me for a while, but they all said the power was too strong to stop. They told me to find a "grizzly bear doctor," a certain kind of medicine man who specializes in or possesses that kind of power.

In the meantime, I had been studying under twelve different medicine men and women who trained me for different kinds of doctoring, rituals, and ceremonies. I also kept up my college education, graduated, and got a job as a professor in Native American studies. My psychic and mystical experiences continued, my apprenticeship continued, my dreams continued, and the vision quests continued at different power centers and under the supervision of different medicine people for different dreams.

Finally, an elderly holy man I had been studying under for years, but not as my main mentor, revealed to me that the grizzly bear was his family medicine. I had suspected that was one of his powers, but out of respect I never asked him. I had told him a lot about my dreams and vision quest experiences and training under other medicine people. Although the subject of the grizzly bear had come up on a number of occasions, he never told me anything about it. One day, after serving as his assistant for the War Dance ceremony, he pulled me aside and asked if I would like to learn about the grizzly bear medicine. I was astounded and delighted. What follows is an account of my vision quest. It is an example of how dreams can lead to visions and visions can determine a medicine man or woman's power:

* * *

Grandfather Sun was just beginning to set behind the mountain when the elderly medicine man slowly walked up to the rock altar. In the distant canyon, a woodpecker drummed. The old man picked up a few willow sticks, gently rubbed them together until they started smoking, and I saw a small flame emerge. Suddenly, the whole western side of the mountain cliff turned a brilliant gold. I was awed, but he continued with his preparations as if unconcerned.

His expression was sober as he reached into the medicine pouch strapped at his side. He pulled out a small handful of tobacco and sacred herbs, faced east with an outstretched hand, and placed his prayer well into the wind. He then turned to the three other cardinal points of the universe and with the same gesture, silently made prayer offerings. Afterwards, he turned toward the sacred mountain with an offering. Then he took the remaining bits of tobacco and carefully sprinkled them into the fire pit. I could barely hear him, yet I knew he was sending an ancient and secret prayer to the highest beings who have been here since the Beginning of Time.

As the old man's song drifted into the sunset, we heard the cry of a golden eagle. It was *talteth*, spiritual messenger and guardian of the sacred high country, medium between humans, spirits, and the Great Creator. We sat by the charred altar and watched the golden eagle circle overhead. He was strong and graceful; higher and higher he flew. I felt an upward pull with him, but the old man broke my trance when he spoke:

"The White People call this mountain Chimney Rock. Our people call it *Hey-ah-klau,* which means Golden Rock, or shrine. It is our most precious power place. It is the home of the mountain spirits, the Little People, the Ancient Ones, and the *wogey.* The *wogey* are what you younger generation of people might consider outer space beings. They enter our natural world through that bowl up there." He pointed toward the golden eagle and the direction it was flying, toward a sky aperture.

"This is our Center of the World. The Great Creator made his final rest here after creating the world. Up there, on that ancient mountain top, is where he sat to meditate, to reflect on the essence of Nature, and to share departing secrets and special powers with the spirits and creatures that live there."

The old man paused to look upward in a sad, reminiscing gaze. Tears rolled down his cheeks. Taking a deep breath, he explained further: "This is the Creator's *tseksel,* a power seat from where he saw everything so pure and beautiful. It was *mer-werk-ser-ger,* there was beauty above him, there was beauty below him, there was beauty all around him. He became one with the power, beauty, and essence of Nature; thus, this place is considered holy."

The Elder sprinkled a few bits of *walthpay* root into the fire. It crackled, its coals glowing brighter, and the smoke encircled us with a medicinal fragrance. "Only those who have been called by a special dream and evaluated by the religious elders can come up here to sit in the Creator's seat," he stated sternly.

"From this high and ancient shrine you can look upon all the other mountains in every direction. To the east," he said excitedly, "rises Mount Shasta. To the south are the Trinity Alps of the Hupa and Wintun Indians. To the west you will see the whale-shaped mountain we call Doctor Rock. That is where auntie Fanny Flounder got her final and most powerful doctor pains. Over there to the north is Sawtooth Mountain; Bigfoot lives on that ridge. Directly in front of you is Chimney Rock, home of the respected grizzly bear, the wolves, the flickerbird, the white deer, and occasionally the golden eagle. Up there, in the very middle of the sky bowl, is the doorway to the unknown and cosmic illumination."

As I listened to his description of the shrine, my mind drifted back a few weeks, and I thought of my training. I had heard Elders talk around the ceremonial dance fires at night, about legendary men who in earlier times embarked upon power quests. Some had encountered large water serpents while swimming in alpine lakes for bravery medicine. Others had wrestled Bigfoot or been tormented by "wild people and woods devils"; some had even encountered a giant two-headed snake. I shuddered, wondering what was waiting for me.

I knew it was a sacrilege to enter the sacred high country without the proper preparation, cleansing, and calling. I had fasted, purified myself in the sacred sweat lodge, and hiked the rugged mountain trails to prepare for this special moment. Ten days of fasting without food and water is a very long time. The arduous hike up almost killed me. The hot sun, the lack of food and water, and the altitude made me delirious.

The old man broke the silence with a high-pitched yell, hollering, "Hey, wogey" four times and clapping his hands. He stood intently as if waiting for a response; we heard the echo, or at least I thought it was an echo.

He sat down, stared piercingly into my eyes, as if trying to read my mind, and spoke. "A person must earn the right to be here, through much suffering and sacrifice, in this life and from a cycle of past lives, to qualify for the calling. It comes through a special dream. The sacred mountain calls you here. One cannot lie about such a dream. You know, the Elders have a way of seeing the truth. If one does receive the dream, he must follow it precisely, forthrightly, and respectfully; he cannot ignore it. Dreams are powerful; they can even destroy a man if he is not properly guided."

He reached for a few more boughs of fir and wood, said a short prayer to each piece, then gracefully placed them into the fire pit. The smoke from the fragrant fir boughs would rid us of human scent. From a small leather bag he pulled a tubular-shaped pipe and tobacco pouch. After packing the pipe with tobacco he offered it to the sacred mountain, then lit it with a coal he casually took from the hot fire with his bare hand. He puffed on the pipe a number of times with his eyes half closed, then handed it over to me. The tobacco was strong; I couldn't help but choke a little while he laughed. "That's the wild tobacco," he said. "You won't find that in a store. It will give you the strength you need."

I carefully handed the pipe back to him. I couldn't hold it; it made me nervous. My hands got hot, and an electrical current ran up my arm as I tried praying with the pipe. He took it and slapped it ten times, emptying the ashes into the fire. After murmuring a few words under his breath, he turned and said, "Here, at the very top of the golden stairs, on the ancient golden altar, with a rare golden eagle and the blessings of a golden Sun, the most powerful Indian doctors and ceremonial headmen have come to be ordained. There are a few in the past who tried it up here on their own without proper preparation and guidance. They always failed. Some of them cheated in their training and it cost them their lives. And there have been others who came up here in quest of bad power. They spent many years in pain, sickness, and torment as payment for their stupidity and sacrilege. It is one of the laws humans have to obey. The Universe with all its wonder and glory is subject to a definite set of Laws as established by the Creator in the Beginning."

The Elder tenderly broke apart the sacred angelica root and continued praying. The Sun had set; the eagle was gone. The hot summer wind had been replaced by a cool mountain breeze. Chimney Rock turned into a dark silhouette against the evening sky. I began to notice a particular bright star in the west which pulsated with a rhythmic humming. It changed color—white, red, blue, purple, and suddenly gold.

The moon was rising from the east over smoke-colored mountains. I felt an unusual vibration that became almost unbearable. I turned my head away from the hypnotic sparkling of the evening star to offer my tobacco to the moon.

Earlier, I had made prayers to the sun. The offering was obviously accepted because the Creator had sent a positive omen of the highest caliber; the golden eagle. Now this extraordinary vision at sunset was the answer we had been waiting for. However, it needed to be verified and balanced by the powers of the night. This exemplified another law, the Law of Cosmic Duality, that everything has two sides: day and night, physical and spiritual, matter and energy, life and death. To achieve harmony, the duality must be properly balanced, a concept the Yurok Indians call *wogi*.

The moon was fully illuminated. It was pure gold, remarkably the same color as the sun at sunset. It vibrated, producing a profound humming sensation that caused me to tremble. I could feel power surging through me to the point where I could not control a sudden onset of convulsions. I was just beginning to lose consciousness when the old man quickly grabbed me by the head and made me sit down next to him. He then spit into his hands and smeared grease from the angelica roots over my face, chest, and arms. He told me to hold on to my pipe and warned, "No matter what happens, don't drop it." In an instant, the sensation ended just as abruptly as it had started.

The Elder remarked: "I almost lost you there for a

moment. Man, are you in for it. Just wait until you get on the very top of the rock. No telling what will happen to you then. Here, sit by the fire and smoke. Take it deep into your lungs and talk to that tobacco. Let it penetrate your entire body and calm you down. We've got a long night ahead of us, and there is more yet to come. *Skuyeni*, this is good."

He started praying again, carefully talking to the spirit of the fire, the spirits of the mountains, and the Great Creator. Then he turned to me with a warning: "Mountains have their own kind of personality and power. A person must know exactly how to introduce himself to each mountain, or he could get hurt. The mountain also has its own family of spirits that serve as guardians. If they don't accept you, you're in real trouble. I've seen some of my friends get hurt and even die over the years because they didn't do right up there. So we have to be careful and follow the traditional custom and laws."

The old man paused, sprinkled more tobacco on the fire, prayed again, looked up into the night sky at a passing meteor, then continued, "See, there's my agreement." We watched a shooting star pass rapidly over the mountain into the void. He said, "I've watched you carefully all these years. I wanted to help you a long time ago, but I knew you weren't ready. I saw how you suffered, sacrificed, faltered, and even succeeded. I heard the gossip, rumors, and lies about you around the Indian community; it was all jealousy. However, I also took pride in seeing how well you tempered the ridicule; that is what made you different from the other people. It is all part of the tests to temper your spirit, small but important obstacles to be overcome before you could qualify for the honor to be here now, in this holy place. However, your tests are not over yet; there is more waiting ahead." He burned some *walthpay* roots in the fire, then loaded his pipe, and again took a small, hot coal from the altar to light his pipe. In a religious way he blew smoke on me several times and said: *"Kimoleni-torquay-et, let-mo"* (all bad things, all sickness, all impurity leave this man).

He began to growl like a bear while looking intently at the mountain top. He drew ten long breaths from his tubular pipe, blew them at Chimney Rock, talked to it in the Native language for a long time, then started singing his grizzly bear song. It was the same song taught to him by his father, who learned it from his grandfather, who learned it from his great-grandfather. He said they had learned it from the doctor spirits and animal guardian who originally inhabited Chimney Rock: the famous grizzly bear. Thus he began the *remopho*, the doctor-making song, or what some of the Native people call the "Kick Dance."

With his cane in one hand, golden eagle feathers in the other, and tears in his eyes, he danced like an old bear around the fire. Even at the age of eighty-four, he was still full of stamina and spirit. It must have been all those former years of spiritual training that gave him the remarkable strength to keep going. Obviously he was right at home in this rough and rugged high country; it was part of him and he was part of it, and everything around us knew it.

My thoughts were interrupted by the power of his song. Four times he sang the grizzly bear formula:

> *Hi-ya-wa-nawa*
> *Hi-ya-wa-nawa*
> *Hay-ah-klau-ni-wo*
> *Neek-wich-so-ney-o*
> *Hin-no-wa*.

To the four winds he offered his tobacco and smoke, to the four corners of the Universe he prayed, and four times he cried out loud to the *wogey*. While he did his ceremony, I thought seriously about the symbolism.

Although ten is normally considered the holy number for the Native people in northwestern California, the number four is also sacred; it is symbolically considered *wogi* by the *Tal*. While ten is an unfolding of unity, four is a quaternity. It is one of the oldest symbols in the world and can be found within all cultures as a universal archetype. For example, Nature is held together by four different forces; there are four sacred directions; there are four basic elements: air, fire, earth, and water; there are four races of humankind: red, yellow, black, and white; there are four seasons; and as humans we have four stages of life. A good medicine man has at least four visions and is given at least four different powers to work with in curing. There are even four corners on Chimney Rock, just like the four-cornered fire pit in the *wogel-ur-girk,* the sacred sweat lodge.

As the Elder sat down by the fire to feast, he continued talking about spiritual matters. "Well, soon we will see if you can become fully qualified as a *mer-werk-ser-gerth.* You have gone through three important phases during your ten years of *hoh-kep* (doctor training). This is your fourth. The apprenticeship helped you to become a seer, ritual leader, and doctor. But you will not be complete until you have been accepted on this particular mountain. If you succeed, you will be considered a true spiritual person of the highest order." He looked me straight in the eyes, paused as if to let the impact of his statement penetrate my soul, then talked some more about the process.

"Now you will be given the rare opportunity to experience *mer-werk-ser-ger.* It is something that really cannot be explained. To be understood, it must be experienced; it is too sacred even to put into words. If you make the proper connection with *Was-en-ow-kay-gey,* you will be complete; but if you fail in your attempt, you could die, or even disappear forever from the face of the earth. Think it over carefully to be sure you want to go through with it. I'm getting old and tired; this will be my last time up here, understand?"

I listened to the soft words of my mentor and seriously pondered the situation. I was tired, hungry, and exhausted. I looked up at the enormous rock in front of us and wondered if I would be able to muster enough strength to force myself to the center top of the ancient shrine. One slip and I could easily fall to my death. I shook with a sudden chill of fear.

It wasn't the thought of dying that made me so afraid; it was something quite difficult to explain. It was a certain gut-sick feeling you can get when you are about to encounter the vast, mysterious, unknown. I had already learned how to deal with death and dying, perhaps as a prerequisite to this coming ordeal. Death itself is nothing to fear; it is the circumstance which leads to the climax of death that is terrifying.

I looked up at the familiar ridge behind Chimney Rock, and the pieces of the puzzle finally came together. All the past dreams, the repeated visions in the sweat lodge, the high mountains, the old trail, the steep canyon and deep gorge, the old man standing behind me singing the grizzly bear song, and now the ordeal ahead. Then it dawned on me. I had been here before many years ago in a dream, while lying in a coma in a hospital 3000 miles away! And my encounter with destiny, and with that rapacious phantom, was not yet completed.

As fear rushed through my body, my thoughts were suddenly interrupted by the elderly headman's actions. He was studying the position of the stars, as if looking for an omen, and quietly singing. Then he turned his eyes toward Chimney Rock, ended his song, and beckoned. "Well, it's time to get ready."

"What's next?" I responded, apprehensively.

"Up there," he said, "on the shrine."

I was taken by surprise. I thought we were going to stay up all night, sing Kick Dance songs, make our prayers stronger, and after the sunrise ceremony I would start the difficult climb.

"The moon is at its apex. It is about 12:00 midnight," he said. "Time to sing the trail song and begin your hike to the top. I told you this wouldn't be easy."

"But how am I supposed to see where I'm going?" I grudgingly responded.

"With your eyes, dummy." He chuckled.

I looked ahead at the ancient trail, barely used for generations. It was fairly distinct at first, but it became less apparent as it meandered into the forest. After that it was obliterated by acres of miserable manzanita brush and darkness. He had to be joking; I thought this must be another test to find out if I am really committed.

"It's not the brush and the piles of sharp rocks that you've got to worry about," he said firmly, "but the hundreds of spirits in the night who live here and guard this sacred place from trespassers. They come in all shapes, sizes, degrees of strength, and supernatural ability. If the *wogey* feel sorry for you, you might make it up on *tsetkel* by around 4:00 in the morning, which is perfect time for the Force to come."

"You're kidding," I said. "How in the world will I be able to see where I am going, much less deal with a multitude of spirits I am not prepared to handle?

He gathered up fir boughs and placed them on the

fire, started singing the trail song, then beckoned me to get smoked.

I was more scared than ever and started to quiver. I thought I felt the ground tremble along with me. Then I heard a high-pitched scream followed by a deep growl. It was far louder and much more powerful than the cry of a mountain lion, often heard in that part of the country at night. I heard the diabolical scream again, this time followed by a horrible smell. I had felt intensely that whatever made the noise was closer. I tried to rationalize it; there aren't supposed to be any grizzly bears left in these mountains, but then again there have been rumors of their return; perhaps it is Bigfoot, but he is only a legend. I felt strongly that whatever it was, it was definitely getting closer. I began to pray for protection. Suddenly, I saw two, huge, savage golden eyes peering out of the forest near the far end of the trail.

The old man simply ignored all the commotion and told me to lie down in the fir boughs. Every once in a while, the ground would shake from the heavy footsteps. I tried to keep vigil the whole time I was being cleansed. "Well, I've done all I can," he said tenderly. "Now you are on your own."

He paused a moment and glanced up at the chimney-shaped silhouette. His eyes sparkled like two stars. Half surrounded by smoke and encased in moonlight, there was a mystical aura about him as he spoke.

"All human beings have a natural desire to be connected with the cosmos. All human beings have the universal right to communicate with creation and the Great Creator. Unfortunately, they seldom make the sacrifice needed to use this right. Rather than going to him, they expect him to come to them in some kind of artificial, man-made church or something. So they sit around in fancy new clothes, with an unclean mind, impure body, contaminated soul, and wait for the Creator to pull up in a Cadillac and bless them all.

"It doesn't work that way. You can't buy the Creator's blessings with money, and you certainly can't qualify for his power and spiritual gifts in an artificial, filthy environment and city. It's a matter of understanding the law, the Law of Respect. That is why he designated certain sacred mountains to be preserved, to be protected, to be used for pilgrimages and for prayer. Up here in the wilderness, in the pristine beauty as it was in the Beginning, is the only place a person can have a chance to meet his Maker. All great spiritual leaders know this truth."

He put some more tobacco in the fire as an offering and looked up toward the sky bowl, then continued, "To fully experience the beauty and essence of Nature, you've got to be completely pure at the time. Very few people ever earn the opportunity to become a *mer-werk-ser-gerth*. So if your timing is off, you will miss a rare fortune. If you are not right in your spiritual ways and commitment, you might die up there, or even disappear off the face of the earth."

I picked up my staff, my medicine bundle, and started walking on the ancient trail which led directly toward those two huge, savage-looking golden eyes still peering so intensely from the dark edge of the forest. I could hear the Elder weeping as we parted company. I was one step beyond.

Although this happened many years ago, I will never forget the vision, the experience, and the power I received. I cannot tell all of it or I could lose it. But I now use that Grizzly bear vision, song, knowledge, and medicine as my main doctor power in healing.

6 ▼ THE TRAINING OF WOMEN
HEALERS: PRESENT AND PAST

▼   ▼   ▼   ▼   ▼   ▼

WE HAVE NATIVE WOMEN HEALERS IN OUR HERITAGE AND culture, but there is not much literature about them compared to books about medicine men. Some of our Native people believe the women are more powerful healers than men. So I think it is appropriate to include some material on their training.

The Yurok, Chilula, and Tolowa Indians live where they have always lived in northwestern California—along the Pacific coast, adjacent to lagoons, lakes, and wild rivers and within the ancient redwood forests. In the early nineteenth century a number of ambitious anthropologists began to conduct research on these small tribal groups whose heritage and culture was rich in spiritual knowledge, tribal myths, healing arts, rituals, and ceremonies.

There were approximately ten Native female doctors in the area when A.L. Kroeber first started his study on the Yurok around the turn of the century. Now there is only one, Tela Starhawk Lake, my wife, a young Yurok-Karuk-Hupa shaman.

What follows are examples of the training of two women from the northwest California Native group who became healers. The first draws on the testimony of Tela Starhawk and includes an interview I conducted with her in preparation for an article in a journal (September, 1981, Trinidad). Tela is a bloodline, hereditary "Indian doctor" from the famous Captain Spott, Fanny Flounder, Nellie Griffin family lineage of the Yurok tribe.

The second example is from the past. It is taken from a classic interview and study by anthropologist A.L. Kroeber of Fanny Flounder, Tela's great-great aunt.

tela starhawk: seeing spirit people

In the following account Tela focuses on psychic encounters, psychogenic phenomena, and shamanistic development:

* * *

You don't wake up one morning and suddenly decide that you want to be an Indian doctor. A person is usually born with it, inherits it, and eventually has to train to cultivate it. In my situation it all started at a very young age. I didn't care much for the other children and lived in my own little world with what you might call imaginary playmates. They were always with me. I hated school and didn't even graduate from high school. It was boring. The other students used to make fun of me and think I was crazy. The teachers and counselors even made me undergo psychiatric evaluation, and a racist judge in Crescent City had me committed to Napa Hospital before my uncle got me out of that mess. But the White people just didn't understand.

It is hard to relate to school, studying, and other students when a person can hear voices, see spirits, and see monsters which the other people can't see or hear. I wanted to be in nature all the time because there I could play with my real friends, the spirit beings and animals.

There is too much to tell, so I will just talk about one psychic experience.

Every time my husband and I went over Bald Hills Road to visit two elderly medicine people who lived at Weitchpec, I would go crazy. Songs started coming in and were too powerful; the songs and voices just wouldn't quit. I wanted to jump out of the car and run down into Redwood Creek Valley. It was like a magnet pulling me. The trees were shaking, the sky was spinning, and the world was full of people, spirit people, of all sizes and shapes. I could hear them singing and see them dancing over by Pasture Rock.

One time it got so bad my husband took me back home and put me in the sweat house. He called his friends over and they sang the *remopho* (doctor-making dance) over me for about five days or so. He said a doctor spirit was calling me from Redwood Creek and I would have to go in there to make a connection with him. I had been fasting on nothing but acorn soup, and he fasted too. We left Trinidad and walked to Orick, then over Bald Hills Road, and down into an ancient village called Noledin. I was tired, hungry, and sore from all those days and nights of dancing at home by the wood heater. It was all I could do to keep hiking. We hiked over prairies, through the woods, and came to a waterfall in the creek. I was shaking all over and couldn't stop it. My husband smoked me with Douglas fir boughs, sang over me, and I went crazy.

Next thing I knew, I was in the water, drowning. I guess I had jumped in the falls before he could grab me. He said he pulled me out of the water and made me sing and dance by the fire.

Later that night a sharp wind hit me, and I passed out. As lightning and thunder cracked overhead, I dreamt about an old woman who lived in the waterfalls. She told me I would get a pain and a song, then I would have to sing it for several days and nights.

Afterwards we decided to go home. I was so weak and sick I could barely climb the steep embankment, high prairies, and small mountainside. We had to stop and rest a lot. My husband said another test would be waiting for me up ahead, but he didn't say what. He just told me not to be scared of rattlesnakes because the prairie would be full of them. He said they were protectors, patrollers, and guardian spirits for the doctor-training grounds.

The sun was very hot. It must have been around noon when I asked him to take a break by the oak tree grove. I figured we could rest up in the shade. He was tired and weak too. I fell asleep for a while and dreamt about a rattlesnake. I can't tell you what she said to me, but I woke up crying and scared. In the dream she had bitten me, and I felt a nauseating pain in my stomach. I was three months pregnant at the time. The bad dream really made me worry about the baby.

My husband calmed me down, burnt some angelica root, and blew smoke over me with it. Then we heard a hawk scream. It came in from the east and circled overhead. My husband talked to it in Indian. He told me I would soon have my test. He said it was a test for strength against fear. He said nobody could be a doctor without first learning how to overcome danger and fear.

Then we started hiking again, and he got ahead of me. After the rest and the dream, I felt even more tired. I could hardly catch my breath because of the heat and thirst. All of a sudden I heard rattlesnakes, and I froze. Directly in my path was a very large snake, coiled with her mouth ready to strike. I didn't know what to do. I shook in fear. I thought about running, but her mouth was arched only two feet from my stomach. I knew if I screamed she would strike.

I could see my husband standing on the hillside, looking down at me. He pulled out his sacred pipe, lit it, and motioned for me to do the same. Very slowly and carefully I pulled it out. I was shaking so that I could barely put in the tobacco and light it, but somehow I managed. The rattlesnake started to uncoil, so I tried to walk around her. But she recoiled and blocked my attempt. Finally I realized that I had to talk to her as one woman to another. So I offered her my tobacco, introduced myself, and asked for permission to pass through her territory. The sacred tobacco had calmed me down enough to confront the danger, and the smoke seemed to hold the rattlesnake spellbound.

Then she talked to me very clearly, just as if it had been a human sitting there. She uncoiled and began to dance around me in a circle. Underneath her were about thirty baby rattlesnakes. They also encircled me, did some kind of dance, and crawled all over my feet as if trying to embrace me. I knew I had been accepted, and I started crying. Then they all slowly filed through the high grass toward Dancing Doctor Rock. I watched them slowly leave, then I walked up to join my husband. He was smiling with pride. He pointed to a golden eagle sitting on the fence post ahead of us. I knew I had passed my test.

This is how the spirits separate the phonies from the real spiritual people who are meant to be doctors.

There is more to it than this, but too much to tell at this time. It is not an easy life to be a doctor. It requires a lot of training. The psychic experiences are very dangerous and real. Things appear physically and then change into a spirit, or vice versa. I guess you call such occurrences psychic phenomena or supernatural, but it is all real. This is just one example of my kind of psychic experience, and native doctor training.

tela starhawk:
bonding with the earth matrix

The following is an interview with Tela in which she discusses her ideas concerning psychic phenomena as they relate to initiation, menses power, and use of ritual for psychological balance.

MEDICINE GRIZZLYBEAR: What is your name and tribal background?

TELA STARHAWK: My name is Tela Donahue Lake. I am thirty years old, and I am a Yurok-Karuk-Hupa-Chilula. My first Indian name was *Keech-wes-ser-it* (Redwood Spider), given to me by my great grandfather, Seely Griffin. The final name given to me by the mountain spirits during the doctor training was kept secret until after my apprenticeship.

MGL: How did you become a shaman at such a young age?

TELA: My great-great-great grandmother, Mrs. Tipsy, was a doctor, and most of my great grandmothers, great aunts, great uncles, great grandfathers were all ceremonial leaders, ritual performers, or medicine people of some kind. So I inherited the knowledge, status, and spiritual power from both sides of the family. When I was a baby, they doctored me in a special way for this position. I guess the old people already knew what I was destined to be. Although some of my brothers and sisters also have the power in them, they were not given a special ritual at a very young age.

As a child I was different from the other children. I could see and hear things that other people couldn't. You would probably call it imaginary playmates, or you would say I was crazy. I could hear songs, see ghosts and spirits, see monsters, and talk to the various creatures in Nature. Or they would talk to me and tell me secrets. And my dreams were very clear. If I wanted to know something I would see it in a dream.

MGL: This unique ability must have made your life fun and interesting.

TELA: No, not really.

MGL: Why not?

TELA: Well, sometimes it was fun, but other times it was difficult because it drove me crazy. It also made my behavior strange around other people, I guess. My younger relatives and friends made fun of me, and when I had to live in the White foster parent homes for a while, I was punished a lot. They (the White foster parents) said I was possessed with the devil, and they would try to beat it out of me. One man even tried to burn it out of me with a hot poker from the fireplace. But I blocked out the pain with my mind. Later on that night I cried, and asked my spiritual friends to help me. I was only seven years old at the time.

MGL: Didn't they even take you to the hospital afterwards?

TELA: No. So I rested up for a few days and then ran away from their home. I was living by myself, cold and starving, for about a week, until one of my older relations found me wandering along the Klamath River.

MGL: What did you do during this time when you ran away? Where did you go?

TELA: I went into the deep redwoods. It was all I could do to walk and sometimes crawl. I spent most of my time crying and trying to doctor myself with leaves, bark, and earth mud. My grandmother taught me how to do this. I would watch her doctor people this way. But I wasn't really alone. The spirits were there with me to help me and tell me what to do. I stayed in a hollow redwood tree with a spider for a friend. This little spider told me not to be afraid.

MGL: Are there other times in your life where you had experiences with pain and suffering?

TELA: Yes, there were many times I got hurt, was in pain, became sick, or went crazy, but it would take a long time to tell you. There are times when I would suddenly have visions, or what you call hallucinate. It was like being two different people in one; it is a kind of craziness.

MGL: Do you think that going crazy or suffering pain is necessary in order to become a doctor?

TELA: Yes, Indian healers are not like White doctors. We don't experiment on animals, birds, and dead or sick people as a means to learn how to cure. We learn everything the hard way, and usually from healing ourselves first. If you can't heal yourself, then you'll never be any good at healing other people. The experience and suffering are very important, all part of the spiritual training.

MGL: What else is involved in the cultural training?

TELA: It all depends on what a woman is meant to be. Some become dreamers, singers, basket-makers, dancers, seers, tracers, Brush Dance medicine women, midwife medicine women, or doctors. A doctor is the highest; it is like being a priest, physician, psychiatrist, and teacher all in one package.

The calling comes through a special dream, sometimes in childhood but usually at puberty. A ghost of a former doctor or medicine woman will come and talk to you in a dream and tell you that you have been chosen for a particular position. At other times different spirits come and talk to you when you are awake or dreaming.

Sometimes the ghost will give you something to eat which will make you sick or give you a pain. In other situations an animal, bird, snake, fish, or whatever will give it to you. This sickness and bad dream will force you to seek doctoring from an older medicine person who in turn will note your condition and help you to cultivate the dream gift.

Then you have to undergo a Kick Dance ceremony for five to ten days. The Kick Dance was originally held in the sacred sweat lodge, but now we have it outside in Nature, or inside a regular house.

Each day I had to gather my wood, cry for help, and fast on acorn soup. I also had to abstain from water, sex, and unclean people, then sweat, sing, and dance until I went into a trance. This is how the psychic power is cooked. The pain will come out in the form of a special, weird-looking vomit. You have to show it to the people and re-swallow it. Afterwards, the young doctor goes to a sacred mountain on a vision quest. This is how she passes her tests and exams from the spirits and the Creator.

I went to *Tsurewa* Doctor Rock, and then I went to Redwood Creek Dancing Doctor Rock. In the winter you train down low along the coast, forests, and rivers. In the summer you go up high into the sacred high country at Doctor Rock and Chimney Rock. Anthropologist Kroeber recorded an example of my great-great-great aunt's training. Her name was Fanny Flounder. Once you get more sets of pains and stronger powers, then you go under an apprentice-ship with an older doctor. (Getting pain and overcoming it leads to initiation as a shaman.) This way you receive confirmation, learn new methods, develop better skills at curing, and gain more knowledge. I trained under Flora Jones, a Wintun doctor, for some of my apprenticeship. For example, I trained for more knowledge and doctor powers in the sacred Black Hills of South Dakota with the Lakota medicine men, and at Chief Mountain in Canada with the Blood and Blackfoot medicine people.

MGL: Does the power always come in a dream, or do you have to actually quest for it?

TELA: It can be either way. Usually the power to become a strong doctor comes unsought in a dream or vision. In later periods of training you actually quest for additional guidance, strength, visions, songs, and power. Female roles other than doctor can be determined by a dream or vision which comes to a young girl in the puberty rite. The Hupa and Chilula have a Flower Dance Ceremony for girls who start their first menses. The Yurok did not have a puberty dance; their ritual was more personal. It is very complicated but basically includes a period of fasting, dreaming, and isolation for five to ten nights.

With the Hupa, for example, a young girl is placed in a special moonlodge which is like an old Indian slab house with the roof removed. They call it a *minkk*. It is similar to their Brush Dance pit, but smaller. The young girl sits in the corner of the pit with her head covered with a deer hide. She faces east and prays for herself, asking the power of the Sun to feel sorry for her and help her to be reborn. A group of dancers come into the pit and sing puberty songs. They have long sticks called clappers which are tapped on the wall. Everyone faces the wall, and nobody looks at the young girl. A medicine woman sits in the center of the pit with a sacred fire and burns herbs and sacred roots. She prays for the young girl while the singers continue singing.

The young girl cannot look at the Sky or anyone. She must concentrate on her condition, a kind of soul-searching, and pray for a vision. At the end of the ten-day ceremony she runs to the river and bathes. She asks the spirit of the water and the Moon to give her strength, protection, long life, and wealth.

Then she returns to the *minkk,* or what is now called a moonhut, and reports directly to the medicine woman. The medicine woman holds up a large abalone shell, and the girl looks into it. Whatever colors she sees in the shell will be reflective of her aura and spirit. Whatever vision she sees in the shell will determine her status in life.

MBL: How is the Yurok culture different?

TELA: The coastal Yurok, *Nererner,* and the river Yurok, *Pulecklau,* did not have an elaborate ritual and dance for puberty. It was more personal and individually oriented, but we still used flowers. Lower class Yurok women bathed at certain places along the Ocean (near a creek) or the River, and upper class Yurok women bathed in a sacred pond, up near the first mountain ridge. Each day she would walk up a special trail, gather her wood, weep, pray for wealth and long life, go up to the pond and bathe, then return back to the moonhut. At this time she is *wes-purawok* which means "she goes to the water to bathe because she is menstruating."

The first day she hikes up once and bathes once, the second day she hikes up twice and bathes twice, until she has hiked ten times for ten days. On the tenth night she stands in the middle of the pond and centers herself between the power of the water and the power of the sky lake, what you call the full moon. Then she prays to Sky Woman and asks for strength, protection, long life, some kind of special gift, and wealth. Afterwards she dives deep into the pond and tries to find a good luck stone. Then she returns to the main house and tells the older women or the medicine women about her dreams, vision, or spirit contact. Thus the tangible and intangible symbols gained from this experience can later serve as psychological resources.

MGL: Is she under any kind of restriction during this ten day period, like the Hupa girls are?

TELA: Yes, she is isolated in the moonhut. This structure is similar to a wickiup. It is upside-down-basket shaped, and made from willow branches. She abstains from water, sex, certain foods, and people in general. She can only travel on the menses path which leads from the hut to her bathing place. She is supposed to fast on acorn soup, dried smoked salmon, and mint-herbal tea. She dreams, concentrates on the meaning of her training, and does a lot of soul-searching.

MGL: Is the ritual still being performed today?

TELA: Hardly at all but a few young girls are doing it in secrecy. Most of the young women today did not have an official puberty rite, so they have developed a substitute which we call a "Moon-time Ceremony."

MGL: What is the Native philosophy behind this pan-Indian ritual? Of what benefit could it be to other modern-day Indians or non-Indians?

TELA: Well, for a woman it is the most important foundation of her health, and a natural cycle for the continuance of good health. When a woman starts her menstrual period, she is being purged by Nature. At this particular time she should be in harmony with the cycles of the Mother Earth and the cosmic forces of the Universe. She therefore should isolate her mind, body, and soul.

It is a sacred time for the woman to diminish herself in order to re-create the totality of herself. It is a time of contemplation, meditation, prayer, and personal atonement. It is an opportunity to center herself and bond herself with the earth matrix. She should thus approach the moontime in a spiritual and respectful manner, with prayers to the Moon.

Since Nature is "purifying" the woman, she will be discharging contaminants, toxins, and negative energy. At the same time, however, the cosmic forces of the Universe will be replenishing her with power. It is for this reason that she must isolate herself and abstain from certain foods, drugs, alcohol, sex, and domestic and cultural duties.

She needs to center herself in order to cultivate her power. She should not disperse or give away this power, because it can be harmful to herself and others. The moontime is a private and personal ceremony with oneself and the earth; as a result it should be mystical, magical, and mysterious. It should not be looked upon with shame or considered punishment.

The moontime can help a woman self-actualize herself; it can help her develop self-reliance; and it can help her to develop intuitive and psychic potentials which are necessary for her survival. Thus it is a time to cultivate her dreams, tap into her unconscious, and synchronize her physical, mental, and spiritual consciousness. The traditional Indian woman considers her moontime to be a mystical experience of enlightenment; hence she approaches the psychic ritual with respect and accountability.

MGL: In the Indian culture the community helps celebrate this new cycle with the young girl, but is the ceremony continued? In other words, after the first puberty rite does the tribe still come out and perform a ceremony over the women?

TELA: No. A ceremony is only performed on her during her first menstrual period. After that she has gained enough knowledge, strength, and experience to continue it on her own, on a more personal basis.

I don't know if Western society can create their own Flower Dance, but maybe they should do something for young girls who start their first menses. Most young girls today go through shock because their society doesn't do anything for them. This is a very special time in every girl's life; it is sacred, and it should therefore be treated in a sacred or spiritual way with a ritual to give it meaning. I'm not saying that White people should copy the Indian religion, but maybe they could relearn their own old rituals, from paganism and druidism.

I once doctored a White woman who had trouble with her female organs. She had not had a period for over six months, and she had a cyst on her ovary. None of the White doctors could find a cure for her problem. So I doctored her and told her what I saw as the basis of her problem. She had been blocking up the flow of her period with a tampon, which caused the negative energy and toxins to kick back into her system. So I told her to lay in the full Moon and to pray to it, to let the light shine on her, and the power of the Moon would return her to balance. I used my herbs and spirits to draw out the negative energy from her body. Then I put her on a self-made moon-time ritual. In just a few months her cycle returned to normal, the cyst went away, and her pimples, head-aches, and cramps cleared up, and her temperamental attitude, frustration, and states of depression disap-peared.

MGL: Do you believe all women need some kind of a ritual for good health and balance?

TELA: Yes, definitely. Menstruation (with PMS) is a natural cycle, and natural cycles require celebration, mentally, physically, and spiritually. Humans must learn to live in balance with the forces, cycles, and rhythms of Nature. Rituals serve to bond us with the earth matrix and keep us in touch with the natural rhythm. When we become disconnected we get sick; we are out of balance.

I told the lady I treated to create her own ritual to

help heal herself. She read some information about European myths and puberty rites which dealt with menstruation in ways similar to our Native religion. And that was what she used as a means to create her own moontime ceremony. So, if women were intelligent enough to do it a long time ago, surely they must be smart enough now to re-create some kind of ceremony to accommodate the special physical and psychological aspects of this important female function.

MGL: Don't you think that ten days is a little unrealistic considering the fact that most women today have to go to work or school?

TELA: Perhaps, but why not compromise? If women can put enough pressure on their society to force industry to give them time off for maternity leave with pay, then why can't they become politically powerful enough to force society to recognize that they should have time off for menstrual re-creation? The long-term effects would benefit everyone.

MGL: Can you suggest an example of a ritual for people who are not Indian or who may not know about their own ancient rituals?

TELA: I'm not suggesting that they go so far as to isolate themselves in a moonhut or moontipi, but they can use some of the old time philosophy and processes. For example, they can abstain from sex, quit eating meat, fast on soups high in potassium, drink lots of herbal teas and fruit juices; they can lie in the moonlight at night and pray for themselves and bathe in cold water for strength instead of hot water.

They can rest, read, meditate, contemplate, practice creative dreaming; decorate a special room in their house for this purpose; share the experience with other women and create a religious cult around the cycle; talk about their female problems with each other in privacy; abstain from work and play during this time; avoid all religious ceremonies and burial rites; or even go so far as to make a special place in their backyard or on someone's farm for a moontime ritual.

They could use an old tub or make a special pond, and bathe in it in privacy, letting the natural forces of Nature aid them. They could stand in the pond or tub, center themselves between two very strong powers, the water and moon, and pray for strength, or seek a vision as they bathe. Thus, during the days a woman is bleeding she can let the poison, organic pollution, and negative energy flow naturally out of her body without interference. Then she can concentrate on the next few days to revitalize or re-energize herself instead of giving her power away through sex, play, work, or social activity. So the bleeding days are used for discharge and the nonbleeding days are used for recharge.

MGL: Well, theoretically it sounds great, but is it really practical? For example, since most women have to work or go to school, they would need time off. Also, what about caring for the children and domestic duties?

TELA: This is where the elderly aunts and grandmothers are valuable. Look how society pushes them off into convalescent homes. Why not adopt a grandparent or an older aunt for this purpose? Why not form female co-ops or use preschools to deal with the problems? This is community spirit. Cooperation is really needed, so why not develop new programs in recreation centers to accommodate the situation? Some women are already using innovative methods to get time off for jazzercise activity. I am sure they can find new ways and means to focus on the most important natural part of their life. Instead of going the entire ten days, they could compromise and have a ritual for five days. It's all a matter of priorities in a person's life. What is more important than good health?

MGL: In conclusion, do you think that ritualization is the key for good health for women today?

TELA: Human beings of all races, both past and present, have always had rituals of some kind. Rituals are natural. All living things in Nature—animals, birds, fish, reptiles, bugs—have their own ritual and ceremony. Without it they could not survive. Why should human beings be different? Aren't they also part of Nature?

Perhaps now, more than any other time in the history of womanhood, we need to bring back some kind of menses rituals for all women. Considering the tremendous amount of female health problems in this nation and the lack of knowledge that has been demonstrated in dealing with them, I believe that the moontime ceremony may be the solution to better health, PMS problems, happiness, and harmony.

fanny flounder: dancing into healing

"Although a shaman's illness is frequently ascribed to the intrusion of malign spirits, such an invasion usually has beneficial consequences. During the often dramatic and painful sequences of combat with evil spirits, neophyte shamans engage in a powerful struggle against the difficult physical and psychological forces that have previously afflicted their lives. That struggle also trains them for future encounters of a similar sort, which they will enact on behalf of others. In fact, the shaman's ability to subdue, control, appease, and direct spirits separates him or her from ordinary individuals, who are victims of these powerful forces." So says Joan Halifax in *Shamanic Voices*.

The following is an example of how a woman became a shaman in northwestern California. Fanny Flounder of the village of *Espeu* told the story to anthropologist A.L. Kroeber at various times. (His report is published in research notes by Robert Spott and A.L. Kroeber titled *Yurok Narratives*, 1942, held by the Lowie Museum of the University of California, Berkeley.)

For several summers [Fanny] danced at *Wogelotek*, on a peak perhaps three miles from *Espeu* north of the creek. It looks over the ocean. Then at last, while she was sleeping here she dreamed she saw the sky rising and blood dripping off its edge. She heard the drops go "ts, ts" as they struck the ocean. She thought it must be *Wes-ona-olego,* where the sky moves up and down, and the blood was hanging from it like icicles. Then she saw a woman standing in a doctor's maple-bark dress with her hair tied like a doctor. Fanny did not know her nor whether she was alive or dead, but thought she must be a doctor. The woman reached up as the edge of the sky went higher and picked off one of the icicles of blood. She said "Here, take it," and she put it into Fanny's mouth. It was icy cold.

Then Fanny knew nothing more. When she came to her senses she found she was in the wash of the breakers on the beach at *Espeu* with several men holding her. They took her back to the sweat house to dance. But she could not: her feet turned under her as if there were no bones in them. Then the men took turns carrying her on their backs and dancing with her. Word was sent to her father and mother, who were spearing salmon on Prairie Creek. But her mother would not come: "She will not be a doctor," she said. Most of Fanny's sisters had become doctors before this. Her mother was a doctor, and her mother's mother also, but her mother had lost faith in her getting the power.

Now, after five days of dancing in the sweat house, she was resting in the house. Then she felt a craving for crabmeat; so an old kinswoman, also a doctor, went along the beach until she found a washed-up claw (the Indians had no way of taking crabs in nets). She brought this back, roasted it in the ashes, and offered it to Fanny. At the first morsel Fanny was nauseated. The old woman said, "Let it come out," and held a basket under her mouth. As soon as she saw the vomit, she cried, *"Eya,"* because she saw the *telogel* in [pain]. Then everyone in *Espeu* heard the cry and came running and sang in the sweat house, and Fanny danced there. She danced with strength as soon as the *telogel* was out of her body. And her mother and father were notified and came as fast as they could. Then her mother said, "Stretch out your hands (as if to reach for the pain) and suck in your saliva like this: hlrr." Fanny did this and at last the pain flew into her again.

This pain was of blood. When she held it in her hands in the spittle in which it was enveloped, you could see the blood dripping between her fingers. When I saw it in later years it was a black *telogel* tipped red at the larger end. This, her first, is also her strongest pair of pains. About it other doctors might say, *"Skui k' etsemin k'el"* (Your pain is good). They say that sort of thing to each other when one doctor has seen a pain in a patient but has been unable to remove it and the next doctor succeeds in sucking it out. The words of Fanny's song when she sucks out blood with her strongest power are: *"Kitelk'el wes, ona-olego' kithonoksem"* (Where the sky moves up and down you are traveling in the air).

Now after a time an old kinsman at *Espeu* was sick in his knee. The other doctors there, who were also his kin, said, "Let the new doctor treat him." Her mother wanted her to undertake it but warned her not to try to sing in curing until she told her to. So she treated the old man without singing; and then she took on other light cases. Altogether she doctored several times before she sang. Then her mother told her to try to sing, and the song came to her of itself.

Next summer she was at the same place on the hill, again dancing for more power. She was stretching out her hands in different directions when she saw a chicken hawk (*tspegyi*) soaring overhead. She became drowsy, lay down, and dreamed. She saw the chicken hawk alight and turn into a person about as tall as a ten-year-old boy, with a marten skin slung on his back. He said, "I saw you and came to help you. Take this." And he reached over his shoulder, took something out of his marten skin, and gave her something which she could not see; but she swallowed it. At once she became unconscious.

At *Espeu* they heard her coming downhill singing. As she ran past the sweat house the people seized her and put her into it, and she danced and came to her senses again. This *telogel* took her less long to learn to control. It is her second strongest pain. After she had taken it out and re-swallowed it she saw that it looked like a dentalium.

Now when she is called on to doctor, if she sees a chicken hawk overhead while she is on her way, she knows she will be able to cure, even if she has not seen the patient; if she does not see a chicken hawk, the case is serious and the patient may die.

The song she got from the chicken hawk is also about the ocean or something near it. When she is not in the trance state she can hardly remember the song, but when in a trance she sings it without knowing it.

When Fanny first told me about her power, she told me only about the chicken hawk. She was saving out how she got her first and strongest pain. That is the way doctors do: they do not give it all away. Nevertheless, other doctors soon find out that a doctor has additional pains, from what they see she can extract and they cannot.

All her other pains came to her later, and are smaller and weaker. She did not have to go to dance at *Wogel-otek* for these; she dreamed and got them at home. That is the way it is with all doctors.

But after she had her first pain it was still necessary for her to "go inland" (*helkau nusoton*). This is like "passing an examination" or proving oneself. This she did only after she had her first pain in and out several times and had it pretty well under control. She went up the peak on which *Wogel-otek* is, but to another part of it on the south side called *Tsektsel otek*. It is so called because there is a *tsektsel* there—one of the seats or semicircular rock walls where the *woge* used to sit down and think. Besides doctors, men can go there to acquire luck. This *tsektsel* is big enough to permit one to sit within it and stretch his legs in any direction. Its open side faces south.

Well, Fanny went up there with her mother, who was also a doctor. She wore her maple-bark dress. She stood aside until her mother had cleaned out the seat and built a fire in front of it. By it her mother laid down a new bark dress for her and a pipe in its case and a *keyem* basket. She told Fanny to put on the new dress and leave the old one. She built herself another little fire a short way off.

Then Fanny stepped into the *tsektsel* and danced just as she had when first seeking power, stretching out her hands in all directions. All that night she did not stop dancing. Occasionally she shouted. When she danced more slowly she clapped her hands together. Her mother had told her, "When you shout you will hear all kinds of things from inland (*helkau*). But say, 'No, I did not come here for that.' Toward morning perhaps you will hear them singing the *remopho* from the mountains. Then say to them, 'That is what I am here for.' "

Then, as the night wore on, she danced harder and harder, and heard the sounds from inland more plainly and shouted, "I wish that when I doctor, any sick person will become well (*wokteu niwa'a soksipa*). I am glad, you will give me the power."

Then at daylight she started straight for the sweat house at *Espeu*. She knew nothing, but the *woge* led her there directly while she sang.

Her mother stayed behind, throwing the ashes from the fire aside, sweeping out the *tsektsel*, and laying Fanny's old dress and basket in the first fork of the nearest tree, tying them against it with two or three strands of the dress so that they would stay there. It was the old basket into which she had spat out her first *telogel* pain that her mother thus put away with her old dress. Fanny's old pipe she laid inside the *tseksel* at the back. Then she slapped her pipe sack five times, poured tobacco into her hand, rubbed it with her other, and blew it off inland toward the mountains. Then she slapped the sack five times more and poured tobacco on the ground before the bowl of Fanny's abandoned pipe. After they lead the novice to the sweat house the *woge* take with them the life of the dress, the basket, and the pipe (*wegwolotsik helkau wesoto*). That is how doctors know that when they are dead they will go into the mountains, and each one while here has to make her path into the mountains. They go inland (*helkau*).

Then Fanny's mother went down to the sweat house at *Espeu*. When Fanny arrived, they were already singing in the sweat house. Others stood outside to keep away any menstruating women, because a woman who was an enemy and menstruating might deliberately come to stand near the sweat house to spoil the new doctor's power. Also, these people outside may be needed to direct the doctor. Sometimes a novice runs straight to the sweat house and dives in through the door headfirst. Others start to wander off and have to be led to the door. Now Fanny had jumped in and was dancing.

The second night, she felt as if she were dancing outdoors, not in the sweat house. When people fell out from the singing to eat or rest, she also rested in the sweat house. She felt weaker and weaker, but did not tell her mother. Then new people from the mouth of the river and up the river came in to sing, and they brought heavy songs (*winoktsenol*). These are slow songs and not meant to be danced to, and her mother had told Fanny not to dance to them, but only to the proper *remopho* songs; but these heavy songs were good, and after them, when they went back to *remopho,* she felt strong again and danced.

Now the rule is that singers must sing four times before passing the song on to the next one; and they go on until the doctor begins to slow down her step and clap her hands; then they stop. On the third song of the first singer Fanny felt all her strength leaving her again. On the fourth song she did not get up until after he was going, and barely managed to stand up. Now most doctors close their eyes when they dance. But on the south corner of the sweat house, where the sky had been showing between the planks, Fanny now saw that from time to time it looked as if it were covered. Then she clapped, the song stopped, she sat right down, and her mother came to her at once. She told her what she had seen. Then the mother told her husband to go outside and look around the south corner of the sweat house. Tipsy looked and looked until he saw a piece of dry salmon stuck into the cracks between the planks. This was *tspurawo uka'm,* menstruant woman's food. He did not touch it, but came back in and told his wife, and she slipped out quietly and removed it while Tipsy told the singer.

Then Fanny danced again and her strength was back. On the third song of the new singer her pain came out and she handled it, both on the *keyem* basket and in her hand, and sucked it back in. Then she was in a trance again, but finished the song and clapped her hands. When they stopped, Fanny's mother whispered to her husband to put an end to the dancing for a while and find out who had secreted the impure salmon, so Tipsy said, "You visitors come to the house and eat." So they all filed out and ate. Meanwhile they summoned the menstruating women, but all made denial. Only one of them would not come, and she was a kinswoman, although a distant one. Then her husband sent a woman to tell her that he would beat her if she did not come. So she came and confessed she had put the impure salmon into the sweat house in order to spoil Fanny's power, but she said she had done it to test how good a doctor she was. Then Fanny's mother told this woman's husband not to beat her, but they made her promise never to do anything like this again.

In the evening they sang for Fanny again in the sweat house. Now everything went fine. She took her pain out four times during the night. In the morning she rested. This is done for ten nights; then the pains are settled and under control for good.

After this, and after her experience with the chicken hawk, Fanny had her roadway to *helkau* established. From now on she could get her dreams and pains in her own house.

7 ▼ APPRENTICESHIP

▼   ▼   ▼   ▼   ▼   ▼

As we can see by the examples of Native women doctors, there are specific steps one must go through in order to become a healer. The process of the shamanistic path is started by inheritance and includes certain trials and tests involving psychic encounters, the influence of dreams which lead to vision-seeking and the calling, evaluation by the Elders, and the actual apprenticeship. Sometimes the process can start all over again due to a new dream, illness, pain, or mystical experience.

The examples used here from the tribes of California are somewhat different from practices of the Native tribal systems of the plains and plateau regions. In addition to training with the California tribes, my wife Tela has also trained and received confirmation from the Lakota, where she did her doctor training in the sacred Sundances, and in some caves located in the sacred Black Hills, along with additional training with the Blood/Blackfeet Indians in Canada. She was guided to these people and sacred places by detailed dreams that she had many years before she even met the people.

In both tribal systems the novice must be constantly "purified" and properly prepared in order to withstand the psychic impact of the vision quest. For example, in my own case, before I could begin my vision quest training and doctoring apprenticeship, I had to get "cleaned up" by the Elders. In northwestern California the Native people use a spiritual approach called "pe-gas-oy" in the Yurok Indian language. It is part of the doctoring ceremony in which you identify the violations you have committed and confess to your transgressions. The medicine man or woman pleads on your behalf to the Great Creator, and the violation is "blown away." Afterwards you are purified by smudging with herbs, or you are placed in the sweat lodge for further purging. The heat, fasting, sweating, abstaining, praying, and use of herbs serve to purify your mind, body, and soul of any contamination; it puts you back in balance with the Universe, and in harmony with yourself. Being out of "balance" can cause you to get sick.

If you as a modern-day person wanted to develop more spiritually, you could use the above knowledge and information. First make a list of the violations you have committed. In the appendix is a list of spiritual violations Northwestern California Indians use. You may want to compile one based on your own religious and ethical background. After listing your violations, for a few days fast, abstain from drugs, sex, and alcohol. Go into a sacred sweat lodge ceremony and confess your violations; but be sure to have the sweat lodge leader of your peers blow over you three times to "blow the violation away," just as the Great Creator calls in the Spirit of the Wind to purify the earth when he wants something cleaned up.

After the dream, the calling, and the vision quest comes the apprenticeship where we are trained in patience and understanding. The training might last two years or two decades depending on the tribal system you are trained in. It also depends on the kind of power you have, what kind of medicine man or woman you will be, and the kind of training you undergo.

I had to train for four years before I was allowed to conduct my first sacred sweat lodge ceremony. For over a decade I had to study, watch, learn, and assist different medicine men and women, who used different approaches and methods of healing, before I was considered qualified to start doctoring on my own. Each time one of my mentors thought I was ready, a different power dream or mystical experience would occur, starting the cycle all over again.

I started out by training in the sweat lodge in the use of dreaming and vision seeking; then I went to the stage of learning how to use plants, trees, and herbs in doctoring; then I was taught how to use my hands and mouth to pull out the pain and sickness; how to transmit healing with my hands; and how to use certain power objects. In later stages I was taught how to see clairvoyantly in order to look into the past, present and future for diagnosis; how to soul-travel to heal long distance or to retrieve lost or captured souls; how to battle against evil powers and forces; how to become a "spiritual" doctor.

The training went day and night, sometimes days on end. I had to learn and memorize certain Native myths and legends, study Nature's symbolic language, and develop the art of omen-reading and interpretation, such as what it means if a hawk flies in, if a snake appears while you are doctoring, if an owl shows up just as you start your ceremony, if a raven or eagle comes; also, what these symbols mean in dreams. I had to learn more of the tribal language while studying under my mentor. I had to learn how to conduct certain rituals and ceremonies, including the proper way to make regalia, how to change the weather, and the ancient prayer formula and medicine-making that went with each ritual or ceremony.

All of the training taught me patience and understanding. There were times, for example, where I had to fast and sit by the sacred fire for hours and days. I was taught to study the fire as I observed my thoughts carefully, watch how it dances and moves, study its changing colors and symbolic meanings, learn how to tolerate its heat, and how to use its hypnotic aura to put myself into deep trances and dreams. I also had to learn how to use the water, different kinds of water, under different kinds of circumstances; how to stare into it until I could actually see the spirit of the water; and how to use it as an ally in healing. I was taught how to "see and hear" the spirits, both good and bad, in order to negotiate their assistance and protection or to get rid of them. All the training in this area required discipline of the mind, body, and soul. I had to learn how to discipline my thoughts and not let my mind wander. I learned to distinguish between fantasy and fact, imagination and reality, sanity and insanity, perceived threat and actual threat, physical and spiritual, life and death.

For example, one time I was heading on my way to the Hoopa Indian Reservation to doctor a person who needed special help. I had just gotten off work and had to take time while driving to prepare myself for the ceremony. As I traveled over the windy, mountain road, fighting the rain and fog, I noticed a redtail hawk come swooping in directly at my car. I actually felt it before I saw it and heard it before I saw it. My conscious mind blocked out the "intuitive-spiritual feeling" and then later the "spiritual hearing" because my mind was occupied with other matters. I had been trained to realize that this was a bad sign; it is not a bad bird, just a bad sign. It means danger. So I automatically slowed my car down, sang a protective prayer song, and watched the road carefully. All of a sudden a huge road plow came from around a blind curve. If I had not seen the hawk as an omen, I would be dead. There have been hundreds of times over the years that a hawk, deer, eagle, bear, raven, snake, bug, cloud, or some other kind of symbolic sign in Nature saved my life or my patient's life. It takes patience and understanding, discipline and a certain amount of madness, to develop this kind of knowledge.

In order to make medicine you must also go crazy. I am talking about the kind of craziness that gets people committed to mental hospitals because their field of reality does not fit Western behavior. The training is arduous, a real strain on the mind, body, emotions, and soul. The extended periods of fasting, the long hikes into high mountains low in oxygen, the extremely hot sweat lodge sessions, and the lack of sleep begin to change the mind. Spending more time in the dream state and less in physical consciousness also begins to change the mind. You start to see and hear things that other people cannot, for instance talking birds and animals, ghosts and spirits. At first you suspect it is only your imagination and look to a friend or your mentor for confirmation. If they don't see or hear it, you begin to think you are crazy. You are afraid to talk about what you are actually seeing and hearing because you don't want people to think you are crazy, so you keep it to yourself at first. But that becomes very lonely; you just can't go around locked up in your own head without communicating to other people. We are social creatures by nature. We learn by social consensus. From the time we are a child our world is described to us; this is a tree, this is a chair, this is a dish, this is a shoe, this is a cloud, this is a rock, etc. If we have doubts about something we ask a parent, a friend, a teacher, a relative. But what about ghosts and spirits and talking creatures when others, except for maybe your shaman mentor, can't see the same phenomena?

When you get hit with the pain and power while standing on a mountain or in the sweat lodge or through a dream, you go crazy. When that force hits your mind-brain complex you begin to hallucinate; you see things that the average person does not even know exist. Sometimes when the power charges through your entire being, it knocks you out, totally unconscious, for hours and even days. That is when you know you are really in trouble and need help. So our Elders have a ceremony to help you "cook" the power and "tame" it. In northwestern California it is called a Kick Dance Ceremony. It lasts from five to ten days and nights. You have to fast, sweat in the sweat lodge or in a ceremonial house, and mentally relive the experience, while the Elders and medicine people sing over you. They start out slowly, then as time progresses move into faster songs. The intent is to work you into a frenzy, a trance-like state, an altered state of consciousness, where you are no longer human but in touch with the spirit. Other tribes use a different approach, mainly the sweat lodge or medicine lodge, but they still sing songs over you, smoke you up with herbs, and coach you until you have tamed the newly acquired power and medicine song.

Afterwards you are given an opportunity to demon-strate your healing power by doctoring someone there who is sick. Once again we see the use of dreams, herbs, and visions as the path to spirituality and becoming a medicine man or woman.

Sometimes, neophytes might not pull out of it; when this happens they either become actually crazy (even to Western standards) or become possessed with the evil power and end up being what we call an "Indian devil" or sorcerer. I never wanted to be a sorcerer, so I kept up my training no matter how dif-ficult it got, no matter how many times I failed.

That is why you must always go to the mountain in order to become a Native healer. At first you start down low, in the sweat lodge, in caves, old trees, or smaller power places. As you keep up your training year after year, you begin to work up to the higher mountains; and in so doing learn how to reach higher states of consciousness, symbolically and spiritually. Each mountain is like a goal to strive toward, but each also has its challenges and obstacles to be over-come. There is something magical and mystical about the mountain; it pulls a medicine person like a mag-net. It haunts you in dreams, it torments you while you are awake. It is constantly on your mind until you get to it, to be tested and receive your gift from the Great Creator. I can understand what Noah, Moses, Job, and Jesus had to go through. The Creator can and does talk to you through anything if he or she so chooses, a rain cloud, a burning bush, a whirlwind, or a high mountain. He talks to our Native American medicine people the same way it has been from the Beginning, for all peoples from all races. He sometimes talks to us through dreams, visions, an eagle, hawk, raven, wolf, coyote, deer, buffalo, snake, rock, bear, lightning and thunder, even a UFO.

It is through this contact and connection with a spirit, with certain powers in Nature, and with the Great Spirit that you get the gift to help and heal others. You learn how to channel and direct this flow of energy and power into the patient during the healing ceremonies. Sometimes the healing connection is very strong, but sometimes it can be weak. It is influenced by a number of variables including our peak days and our low periods. This is another reason why a Native healer must constantly keep up training and get "recharged" in the wilderness and mountains, or strengthen the healing connections by periodically visiting certain power centers and using the sacred sweat lodge. After reading the next chapter where I talk about the healing process, hopefully you will understand what I am trying to share here.

8 ▼ NATIVE HEALING:
ITS PHILOSOPHY AND PRACTICE

▼　　　▼　　　▼　　　▼　　　▼　　　▼

I HAVE DOCTORED PEOPLE FROM ALL WALKS OF LIFE AND
with every kind of sickness. I do not doctor all the
time because it could burn me out. But I have
doctored people for cataracts on their eyes, for blind-
ness, people who had chronic arthritis, broken bones,
torn ligaments; I have doctored people who had cancer, Hodgkins disease, and leukemia; men with prostate gland disorders, women with female organ problems and cysts on their ovaries, children with diseases,
elders whose vital organs such as the gall bladder, kidneys and heart were weakening. And I have handled

less difficult but serious cases such as bug bites, colds, flu, bronchial infections, asthma, food poisoning, cuts, bruises, mental breakdowns, anxiety, nightmares, panic attacks, skin rashes, allergies, and infections. I have dealt with death and dying, possession, and those affected by sorcery. Not everyone was completely healed, but most of them did get healed temporarily, partially, or completely. There were some cases that I just couldn't handle. I had to send the patient to a different medicine person or to a special kind of White doctor. In a lot of cases my doctoring was supplemental because we have all become dependent upon Western medicine for survival. Thus my role has been a combination of medical and religious, part priest, part psychologist, and part physician, but always spiritual in basis.

I have come to the conclusion that nothing is an accident. Every illness, accident, or injury happens for a reason. The most difficult part of "Indian doctoring" is to get at the cause or causes of the problem. I can only talk from my own experience, hence I am sure that someone, somewhere may disagree with me, but in the majority of cases I have handled, the patient's sickness can be directly traced to committing a violation against the natural and spiritual laws, or they may have inherited the violation. This causes the individual to get out of balance, and disharmony causes illness: mentally, physically, emotionally, and spiritually.

In order to make the patient well, we have to take a holistic approach and doctor all parts of the human constitution. The Indian doctor believes that it doesn't matter what tribe, race, nationality, religion, or belief a person has; each one is subject to the Creator's laws and natural laws as established in the Beginning. Unfortunately, most people don't even know the law, but ignorance is no excuse from the law. Some of the laws are similar to what you find in the Bible, but in the Native way it is handed down orally through sacred teachings such as myths or ceremony.

For example, a Whiteman who was married to a Native woman in Alaska came to be doctored. He had chronic osteo-arthritis. He was very crippled and in severe pain. He had been to every kind of Western physician and even a couple of psychologists, but nobody could alleviate the pain or enact a cure. I doctored him, sang and danced on him for three nights, used certain herbs on him for a week, and then purified him in a sacred sweat lodge ceremony. The cause of his illness was simple to diagnose: he had shot and killed large animals such as the bear, buffalo, elk, deer, and moose without proper ritual and agreement. His wife had handled, cooked, served, and eaten the meat while she was on her moontime (menses). That is a violation against the Creator's Law and the spirit of the animal. You may consider it ancient, dogmatic, or simply a Native custom and belief, but it is a reality. In order to get well this man had to confess his violations. The cause had to be identified, he had to admit to the violation, then atone by apologizing and offering tobacco as a form of restitution.

I have handled cases where people's sicknesses were due to all kinds of violations such as killing rattlesnakes without just cause, digging up burying grounds, gathering herbs and roots without a proper prayer and agreement, polluting sacred waters, having sex upon ceremonial grounds, making bad prayers and wishes against others, abusing spiritual knowledge and powers, stealing, tormenting and experimenting on frogs and animals, playing with power or witchcraft, attending funerals while unclean in body and soul and not purifying oneself afterwards; the list can go on. It may be hard for you to accept this, but it is the basis of Native healing.

Sometimes people are in pain because they are being tormented by ghosts, spirits, and forces out of ignorance; they simply entered the abode of a bad spirit while camping, hiking, or partying. There are shadows and forces on this earth who are mischievous; they like nothing better than tormenting human beings. Such entities must be captured and removed, sent back or destroyed before the patient can be made well. There are insane asylums in this country full of people who have become possessed, no matter how the White doctor tries to rationalize and explain it. Sometimes these shadows and forces will cause people to get in accidents to knock them out, and then they steal their soul. If this happens the person will be in a coma. We call that kind of sickness "soul loss." It takes a special kind of power and knowledge to track down the lost soul, fight like a warrior against the shadow or spirit to get it back, then put it back in the body in such a way that the vibratory level will be harmonized. If the vibratory level is not in balance the person can develop certain kinds of side effects that come in the form of other kinds of sicknesses: hearing loss, poor eyesight, skin rash, allergy, or arthritis. That is why our traditional Native people always want a ceremony done on them in the hospital just before and right after surgery; they don't want to take the chance of losing their soul or becoming possessed by a deceased person who is still lingering around the hospital.

examples of doctoring

Perhaps the following examples can demonstrate my point. A middle-aged Lakota college student came to see me and asked for doctoring. For about three days before he came to my house, I kept having tormenting dreams about being drunk and running over an elderly woman. During the day I heard voices talking to me to the point that I was going crazy. It was difficult for me to do my lectures at the university because the voices kept interfering and interrupting my concentration. The students started to notice my behavior, as I would stop in the middle of the lecture, turn around and look, and ask, "What do you want? Who are you?"

After about three days my wife and I decided to

smoke and pray and find out what was going on. The night we planned to talk to our spirits an Indian man came to the house and approached us for a healing. His eyes were very dilated, one hand was twisted up, and he kept looking around in a state of fear while trying to talk to us. He explained that he had been in a mental hospital for over a year and since discharge had been receiving counseling and medication from a psychiatrist. He said: "I keep having these tormenting dreams about dead people. I hear voices in my head a lot. I can't sleep, and I am a nervous wreck. The White doctor said I am paranoid, and he has me taking these pills but it doesn't seem to help. So when I go to see him I just lie about it. I say, sure, it's getting better. I don't have much to offer because I am poor and trying to start college. Will you accept this pack of cigarettes and necklace to doctor me?"

Luckily my wife and I were not under the influence of sex at the time so we could start immediately. During the ceremony we could "see" the cause of this man's problem. He had gotten drunk in the San Francisco Bay area one night, and while driving ran over an elderly woman who was crossing at a dark intersection. The woman died. He spent time in prison for his offense, and he was punishing himself with guilt. He was also being tormented by the deceased woman's ghost and her dead relatives.

We used the power of the wolves on him. We asked him if what we saw was true, and if so would he be willing to confess his actions and beg forgiveness from the woman's ghost. He admitted to his violation, so we asked the Great Creator and the deceased person to forgive him. We built a special fire outside the house and offered a pack of tobacco and some food to the deceased as payment for what the patient had done. In this way, he made restitution.

Then we had the spirit of the wolves and ravens remove the deceased people from the earth plane and send them over to the spirit world where they belong. As a follow-up to the healing, the patient was purged of the Western narcotic medicine and rejuvenated with natural herbs. In addition, it was suggested that he write a letter of apology to the deceased woman's family, asking forgiveness for what he had done, and he was instructed to make restitution to this family by sending them a special gift, something that the patient considered of personal value. He came back a week later looking great. His hand was not bent and crooked anymore, his eyes were clear and straight, and he appeared normal and happy.

In the above example we can see how difficult it is for this form of reality and knowledge to fit Western medical standards, but the Native approach to healing seems to work. Here is another example, not involving an Indian but an Asian.

Some Vietnamese people phoned us and asked for help. It was difficult to understand their broken English, so we asked them to come to the house with a translator. Evidently their cultural belief system is similar to ours, for they brought food, a nice blanket, cigarettes (as a tobacco offering), and a money donation. They said their grandmother was in the hospital dying. She had gone in for gallbladder surgery and had been in a coma for several days. They also said that the White doctors hooked her to a life-support system but did not know what else to do except wait and hope for the best.

Most hospitals will not let us do ceremonies on people without prior agreement and arrangement by the attending physician. We have to give the entire staff an orientation and explanation of what we are trying to do, put up with the often prejudiced attitude, and work around hospital policy. If the patient is a Native American we can stand on PL 95-341, the American Indian Religious Freedom Act, as justification to perform a Native healing. But if the patient is non-Indian it becomes more complicated.

The attending physician agreed to let us do the ceremony, as long as we kept the noise down. We could not burn tobacco or herbs around the patient due to an oxygen apparatus. As a substitute we brought boiled herbs and purified the patient and room by steaming. We used sage for this purpose, and we lightly bathed the patient in sage. We also made four different colored tobacco ties (white, red, yellow, and black) or what we call spiritual flags. These are pieces of cloth with a handful of tobacco placed inside, then tied. They are offered to the four powers of creation, to the higher spirits, and symbolically represent the elements of wind, fire, earth, and water. In this way we made an altar of the patient's bed, used eagle feathers, quartz healing crystals, and other regalia that have specific powers and are connected to specific spirits. We then went outside the hospital and smoked our pipes privately in a lawn area. We prayed and called the spirits in and asked for their help. Our spirits told us that the woman's soul had left the body out of fear and bewilderment. It had gone over to Vietnam because she did not like it here. She wanted to be with her other relatives and in a more familiar environment.

My wife and I meditated, and we asked our spirit guides to help us soul-travel. We contacted the woman's soul wandering around an old graveyard in Vietnam. After some difficult coaching we finally talked her into returning to her children in America who needed her. By the time we came out of our trance and walked up several flights of stairs to the hospital room, the patient was awake and out of her coma. Everyone was excited and happy. A couple days later she was discharged from the hospital.

During the healing I had seen a poisonous snake on the woman in spirit form. I asked her daughter and relatives if the woman had ever killed a snake or been bitten by a snake. They replied that they did not know. I told them we would take it off her because it was the catalyst for her original sickness. Several days later they came for a follow-up visit, and the elderly woman, who could not speak English, told the translator that it was true, she had been bitten by a poisonous snake prior to coming to the United States and had killed it.

Although the above example had a happy ending, I do not want to give the impression that Native healers are miracle workers. There have been times that we could not retrieve the soul. In one particular situation the person did not want to come back from the land of the deceased. He felt he had wasted his time while alive and wanted to go on with whatever was waiting for him in the spirit world. That person was my father. The first time he had a massive brain hemorrhage he was in a coma for over a week before we could bring him back. A year later he was pronounced clinically dead. I went over to the spirit world and tried to convince him to return, but he was adamant in his choice. In another situation, the spirits told my wife and me that they could not help because the person in the coma was being punished. I learned soul-travel doctoring because of the death experiences I had as a child and teenager. I have developed that knowledge and skill further by learning from my mentors, from the spirits, and by practice. But I cannot always do this kind of doctoring because it is very strenuous and dangerous to my own body and mind.

the indian code for living

People often ask me during training workshops and lectures, "Is there some kind of code for living that the Indians used as a spiritual guide in their lives, like the Christians and Jews following the Ten Commandments and Muslims following the Koran? In our belief, a person who commits a sin will be punished by God, and this can cause illness and misfortune."

My response to this question is simple and affirmative but needs some explanation. For example, our Native tribal systems did not have a written holy book to guide people in their lives, but they did live by what we call Indian custom and laws, natural laws, and the Creator's Laws. Spiritual guidance, morals, ethics, and a code for living can be found in tribal myths, legends, and "Coyote stories" and were told to the people by medicine men and women during rituals and ceremonies.

Some of these spiritual laws have been discussed in previous chapters of this book, but we need to understand there were over 300 different tribes in the United States. As a consequence, some of the beliefs, customs, and spiritual laws may be the same for all, but in other tribal systems it was different. One example that is common to all Native people around the world concerns the belief (or understanding) that it is against the Creator's Law to hunt, fish, and gather natural resource materials without proper prayer, or unjustifiably to kill our relations in nature, such as deer, elk, moose, bear, wolf, coyote, shark, porpoise, otter, beaver, bird, salmon, snake, spider, tree, plant. There is also a common belief and law among Native people concerning behavior around burial grounds, ceremonial grounds, sacred sites, religious dances, and rituals. In some tribes rape was not tolerated, but in most tribes polygamy was naturally accepted. Death by accidental killing had to be compensated with payment of some kind while deliberate murder required punishment. Stealing within the tribal system was not tolerated, while stealing from enemy tribes was considered honorable. The Indian belief was that most of the sins related to sickness, as you understand it, were in the form of violating laws against Nature.

doctoring ceremonies

The Creator's Laws were normally taught and reinforced to the Native people during rituals, sacred dances, ceremonies, and during "doctoring" when a person became sick. This is another reason why medicine people are so important to a society; they serve as keepers of the faith and religion and try to promote spirituality, good health, and good living for the people. Anyone who violated the law could approach a medicine man or woman for assistance, confession, and prayer. Sometimes the Native people used the sacred sweat lodge for this purpose: they would confess their sins and violations while in the sweat lodge, then purify their mind, body, and soul. Originally, almost all tribes used confession to deal with transgressions. Today, a lot of Native people have either forgotten their original ways or have not been taught the customs and laws; some follow Christianity. But it is not too late to learn.

Most doctoring ceremonies employed by healers in northwestern California lasted three to four days and nights. The patient's family was usually included in the healing session, and the patient was encouraged to become directly involved in his or her own healing process. Ingredients of the ceremony required the smoking of a pipe as a means to communicate with the Great Creator and powers of the Universe. The pipe was also used as a means to summon the shaman's spirit allies; in this sense it served as a "key to the spirit world" where a host of supernatural aids and higher powers wait to be called upon for service. Other doctor's tools included a staff, sometimes flickerbird feathers, an eagle wing, a bowl of water, and various herbs used for invocation and smudging. For example, pepperwood leaves are burned to ward off evil powers and forces, angelica roots are burned to "attract and feed the good spirits," and food in the form of acorn meal was offered to feed ancestral spirits, who also offered their healing advice and assistance to the ceremony. The herbal smoke, songs, dancing, and ecstatic environment help the medicine man or woman achieve an altered state of consciousness, a trance-like state needed to activate innate psychic abilities and clairvoyant powers.

Powers such as ESP, clairaudience, clairvoyance, telepathy, soul-travel, telekinesis, and "energy transfer healing" all served as spiritual tools. The shaman did not need an X-ray machine to diagnose various forms of human injury and sickness because he or she could see the problem with clairvoyance; the shaman did not need Kirlian photography to verify the presence of ghosts and the human aura because he or she could "see" and "feel" the phenomena, and "communicate" with them. Thus narcotic herbs were rarely needed for self-induced visions and drug psychotherapy, but the same Native healer did have good knowledge in the use of special herbs for pathology.

9 ▼ PSYCHIC PHENOMENA AND SYMBOLISM IN NATIVE HEALING

▼   ▼   ▼   ▼   ▼   ▼

DURING MY TEN-YEAR APPRENTICESHIP AND TEN-YEAR PRAC-
tice as a Native healer, and as a result of research
among the Yurok, Wintun, and Karuk on the effects
of stress, I had the opportunity to study beliefs re-
garding sorcery, psychic phenomena, and omens. For
some time, I have emphasized the need for a more
holistic approach to Native health; I will now go a
step further and say there is a vital need for modern
health practitioners to recognize the potential impact
of sorcery and psychic phenomena.

During my personal research on Native patients

and their families being treated for a variety of conditions at the Mad River, the General, and St. Joseph's hospitals in Humboldt County, I noted that out of twenty case studies involving patient deaths, at least seventeen persons claim to have seen natural symbols (omens) appear immediately prior to a patient's operation. Ten physicians openly admitted the sudden and strange appearance of certain animals, birds, snakes, toads, or bugs, either in or near a patient's room prior to surgery. Four of the seven physicians interviewed remember having bad dreams prior to the death of their patients. One local psychiatrist and three psychotherapists who are involved with some of the same Native patients also admit that omens appeared during psychoanalysis. For example, Dr. Tom MacFarlane relates: "Now that I think about it, this one patient complained about having bad dreams of dead people. While we were discussing it in my office and attempting to analyze the dream, a bunch of blowflies suddenly flew into the office. I found it strange but simply dismissed it as a coincidence. I do remember, however, that the Indian patient became disturbed about those large flies for some personal reason."

Generally, White physicians do not believe in phenomena such as this. As a result, in a number of the cases I have observed over several years, the symbols and psychic phenomena associated with sorcery were apparent but ignored. Unfortunately, because those involved failed to recognize or refused to acknowledge the potential and presence of psychic power, a considerable number of patients may have died or suffered further decline in health, hence requiring a longer period of doctoring.

the power of symbols

Native cultures are predicated on a whole system of symbols which are not well known to Western medicine. However, these should be identified during the diagnosis and treatment of Native patients. For example, in most Native cultures the owl represents a bad omen. The Yurok, Hupa, Tolowa, and Karuk believe that "Indian devils" (sorcerers) use the power of the owl as an ally to harm their intended victims. Other tribes I came into contact with across the nation have similar understanding. Because the owl symbolically represents sickness, evil, death, or sorcery, the traditional Native patient relates to this symbol as a bad sign. Whether it appears in a dream or manifests physically, this symbol can promote fear in the traditional Native person and is perceived as a psychological and spiritual threat. Certainly both perceived threats and actual threats can cause stress, and stress can cause a host of psychological and physical problems. The continual appearance of this negative symbol in the Native person's dreams, or the continual physical appearance of an owl around the Native person's residence, can be either the actual cause of sickness (via sorcery) or the psychic basis of sickness.

Symbols are a kind of energy, and energy can

change form; it can be positive or negative, tangible or intangible, seen or unseen. Negative symbols and negative energy (whether seen or unseen) can produce stress upon an organism, and too much stress can cause mental, physical, and spiritual (psychic) illness. The Native person who fears a particular symbol, the owl for example, is under stress. Thus in one way or another that owl is related to the patient's sickness.

While it may be difficult for Western practitioners to accept Native concepts of sorcery, the appearance of psychic phenomena clearly causes a real form of stress and should be handled appropriately. Furthermore, the patient's belief system about dreams and omens can provide a key to identifying the potential cause(s) of the patient's illness. The doctor's awareness of the psychic symbols in a patient's dreams and of certain psychic phenomena during diagnosis and treatment might provide the clue for resolving the problem and hence curing the illness.

It is easy to understand how a patient who believes in sorcery and spirit phenomena can be mentally affected by them, but what about Native and non-Native people who do not subscribe to the Native belief system? Can their mental problems and illnesses be attributed to sorcery? Is there some other cause which might actually be considered a form of psychic phenomena? Or is the illness simply physical in origin? My observations indicate that while the Western patient may not have the same belief system, the same understanding of natural symbols, or a similar set of archetypes, he or she still can and often does respond unconsciously to such negative symbols. Why? As Jung relates: "At the deeper levels of their unconscious they [modern Western people] too are an archaic being."

ritual relieves stress

Very little has been done in modern medical science to consider how psychic phenomena are related to stress. I believe the Native healer and his or her knowledge in this area has much to offer Western medicine.

A classic example to demonstrate this point involves a patient by the name of Anna O., whose case was associated with Joseph Breuer and Sigmund Freud. By means of hypnosis, Breuer was able to trace the cause of his patient's paralysis to an evening when she fell asleep at the bedside of her dying father. "She dreamt of a large, black snake moving toward him, but when she tried to lift her arm to drive the snake away, she found it paralyzed." Using a Western approach, Breuer attributed the paralysis to the patient's unconscious guilt over feeling resentful of her bedside duties. (P. Robinson, "Reanalyzing Anna O. a Century after the Talking Cure," *Psychology Today,* August 1984)

The Native shaman would consider the snake as the real culprit and the guilt feelings secondary. Removal of the snake, symbolically and psychically, would be the primary objective of the shaman's approach. Purification of the patient to prevent a relapse (return of the snake) would complete the therapeutic process. I believe that Western practitioners could learn a lot from the Native healer's approach to healing, especially about the physical and psychic realms of symbolism.

native symbols and stress

Let me give you an example of how a Native healer and spiritual/psychic knowledge worked as a support system to a Native patient, in collaboration with a White physician, in a hospital setting.

A local physician who specializes in natural childbirth was notified that his patient was ill at the hospital. He met with her in the emergency ward and diagnosed her condition as acute toxemia, a serious condition caused by toxins circulating in the blood. She was within one week of her expected delivery date. The potential danger of extreme high blood pressure left only two choices: either induce labor or perform a Cesarean operation. The patient did not want a "C-section" and requested that she be allowed to have a Native midwife "make a ceremony on her in the labor room for protection and spiritual assistance." The doctor agreed. After labor was induced, the patient's cervix stayed at two centimeters for three hours, and the doctor decided to go home and rest until it dilated to eight centimeters. In the meantime, as the patient was monitored by the nurse, the patient complained of seeing "bad omens" in her hospital room. Evidently, a large spider had fallen from the ceiling upon the patient's stomach, and a toad was found in a dark corner of the room.

Sometime later the physician called to report that he was ill and a substitute might have to be found. He indicated that he had suddenly felt an onset of flu-like symptoms. He came into the hospital for treatment. Lab tests were conducted, and an examination administered, but no cause for the sudden sickness could be determined.

The patient's husband, who had been restricted to a sacred sweat lodge at this time, unexpectedly appeared at the hospital and said, "I had a vision that my wife, the baby, and her doctor were under attack by witchcraft. How are they doing?"

The husband was told that his wife was under severe stress, had toxemia, and that a Cesarean operation now seemed imminent. The husband immediately instructed the Native midwife to use a different ceremony, incorporate a new prayer formula, and use a different set of power and religious objects. He also had the physician paged.

The physician and husband met in the lobby and discussed the situation. The physician remarked, "You know, I was fine until I heard the chickens screaming in back of my house just around sunset. I went outside to see what was going on, and all of a sudden a large owl swooped down as if to attack me.

Now, that is uncanny! What does that mean according to your Indian belief system?"

The husband and the midwife doctored the White doctor. They smoked him up with cedar, prayed over him with a special formula and song, and then had him drink an herbal concoction of water, wormwood plant, and pepperwood (Umbellularia californica) leaves. The physician purged himself, slept for an hour, bathed in cold water, and came back on the job completely renewed. The baby was delivered vaginally with no side effects.

The physician could not believe what was actually happening, but at least he was willing to utilize the Native perspective, knowledge, and rituals as a means to help himself and the patient. He claims that he did not believe in sorcery, but admits that "something psychic was definitely going on which just can't be explained."

Was the sudden sickness of the doctor a reaction to stress and overwork? Was the attack by an owl just a figment of his imagination, or was it a manifestation of the negative symbols in his own subconscious? Was the appearance of an owl just coincidence, or could it be a case of "synchronicity," as Carl Jung might consider it? Perhaps sorcery was being employed, but the doctor's modern, Western-oriented mind refused to recognize it.

There is one very important point to consider here, regardless of anyone's perspective about this case; a variety of symbols appeared physically and psychically to warn all those who were involved in the childbirth process. A ritual was used to rid the environment of all these negative symbols, symbols that were stress-producing in the sense that they were perceived as threatening. When the threat had been removed, the stress was eliminated, and a positive healing effect emerged.

a native view of panic disorder:

Dr. Abby Fryer, a researcher-psychiatrist at Columbia University and co-director of the Anxiety Disorders Clinic at the New York State Psychiatric Institute in Manhattan, has been conducting some interesting studies on an illness called panic disorder. Panic attack victims typically experience a sudden and inexplicable wave of terror, often accompanied by such symptoms as breathing difficulty, pain or a feeling of tightness in the chest, palpitations, sweating, shaking, dizziness; and perhaps most frightening of all, a sense of nonreality, of losing control, of becoming schizo-phrenic, and/or dying. Dr. Fryer discovered that some patients, usually in their late forties, experience such attacks after exercise. Other doctors suspect that these individuals produce more than the usual amount of lactic acid. But the actual cause of these attacks is not understood. Most Western researchers believe it is a physiological illness.

The most common treatment used to alleviate the panic syndrome is tricyclic antidepressants such as imipramine, which is supposedly not habit-forming.

The problem with this syndrome is the recurrence of attacks, with the frequent eventual result that most victims begin to develop paranoia and abnormal fear of being left alone, of flying, of riding in elevators, and so forth. There is a possibility that it might be linked to stroke or be the catalyst for a stroke.

Charlie Thom (Red Hawk), a Karuk sweat lodge-steam doctor, has had to deal with a number of such cases. He indicates that this illness is a prime example of what he calls the "shadow syndrome." Thom says nature is full of good and bad spirits. One of these is a shadow type "force" which lives in various bogs, woods, and swamp areas. It can be seen by the human eye if one catches a side-glimpse of it darting suddenly across the glade or hiding behind trees and brush. This "shadow" often follows people home and torments them by causing poltergeist types of activity: opening doors, rattling windows, etc. Periodically, it even attacks by jumping full force onto the victim's chest. It is often seen as a shadowy figure darting across the room, but most people simply dismiss it as a figment of their imagination. Thom further explains that the shadow comes in two forms: human or a large cat. In an interview I had with him he explained:

"I have had to doctor a number of people for this illness. This is what White people would probably call an example of psychic phenomena. The shadow is alive, it is real, it is a force which lives in Nature and has no other function than to torment and bother human beings. I don't really know why it will attack some people and ignore others, but I think it likes to prey on those who have a weak aura; or people who are emotionally or mentally weak and under some kind of stress. These shadow-spirits are very territorial, so sometimes they will just attack humans because we are in their territory. For example, a man in Eureka went to play golf and came under attack. He went to all kinds of White doctors who thought this man was having a heart attack or something. The golf course was built in a bad place and people shouldn't go there, but I guess they don't know any better.

"This man eventually went to seek counseling from a psychotherapist because his family doctor thought the sickness was caused by stress. But the psychotherapist could not cure the illness, so the patient came to a spiritual-psychic gathering at the Stewart Mineral Springs, near Mount Shasta. The patient thought he could find an alternative health cure, and that is how I met him.

"I took the patient into the sacred sweat lodge ceremony, used spiritual power to fight off the 'shadow' and send it back to where it came from. Then I steamed the patient with herbs to purify his mind, body, and soul.

"I also made up some herbal medicine and mineral water to complete the doctoring; then I told the patient to use this sacred *keeswoof* root (angelica ssp.), to pray with in the event the shadow should return. Teaching the patient how to use a ritual to deal with his problem gives him better confidence and control over his own life. The power of the herb can be smelled and is used as an incense offering to the good spirits; it wards off evil powers.

"It takes power and knowledge to fight unseen or supernatural forces. Sometimes words are just not enough; the patient must have something tangible and special to use and believe in, especially in matters involving intangible causes. I saw this patient a year later, and he said he had only had one more slight occurrence of the problem. He used my medicine and ritual and got completely well."

This is a case some might identify as panic disorder or as a psychiatric case, but it was perceived by the shaman as caused by psychic phenomena. Could the shamans in this situation be right and the hypotheses of psychiatrists and physicians wrong?

autism: working with the ``little people''

Consider also such psychopathological cases as autism, juvenile schizophrenia, and childhood mental retardation. Are such cases simply a matter of physiological and/or socio-psychological disorders, or could they be caused by psychic phenomena?

Have you seen the movie entitled *The Entity*, which was supposedly based upon a true story? Western practitioners were not capable of dealing with such a psychic "force" as it portrays. Is it possible that a child diagnosed by Western doctors as autistic could actually be possessed by an evil spirit? My wife, Tela Starhawk Lake, tells of a case she treated:

"I don't know what that word [autistic] means, but I did doctor an eight-year-old Indian girl who was supposed to have that kind of sickness. She was a distant relative from Crescent City. The mother of this child came down to visit me with her little girl. The mother said her little girl was retarded; nobody could get her to talk. The mother said the White doctors called the sickness autism. Evidently the child had been like this for two years and was receiving some kind of special treatment at a school where doctors, counselors, teachers, and other little children all worked together on the mental problems of the children.

"This little girl did act like she was retarded. What I mean is the way she behaved: withdrawn and glassy-eyed, as if in a deep trance, no kind of verbal, physical, or mental response. She would run over into a corner and try to hide from other people. She wouldn't even dress herself, she frequently messed her pants, and usually she had to be fed. No matter what anyone did, she would not talk or play; she frequently stared off into space. She shook in fear if anyone raised their voice in anger, and she was very afraid of adult men.

"I agreed to help this little girl because I felt sorry for her. I could hear her talking [by clairaudience] to herself and to imaginary playmates in her own head. So, that night I did a healing ceremony. I could see the cause of her problem was simple; this little girl was locked in a spiritual dimension under the protective custody of the Little People. Physically she was here, in the physical world, but mentally she was in the unseen world, the spiritual world. She ran into that dimension by soul-travel as an escape from the social-cultural world where she had been verbally, mentally, and sexually abused. The mother, who was a three-time divorcee, was part of the original problem. An environment of drinking, drugs, poverty, parental fighting, and neglect had forced that little girl to seek help and protection elsewhere. The Little People, the child's imaginary playmates, were in complete control of the child's mind and soul. The Little People are real spirits. For those of us who can see such things, this so-called fantasy was a reality, but the parent and the doctors could not 'see' [in a clairvoyant way]; hence they could not reach this child mentally."

Tela explained that this case was complex, for several reasons. First of all, the problem started from a social-cultural situation which forced the child to seek protection and escape in a spiritual and mental way; that is, she had to find a means to get out of her physical predicament. She was too young and afraid to run away from home, so she sought escape through fantasy and imagination. The shaman further related that children at this age are pure, and thus prone to spiritual (psychic) awareness and experiences. The constant abuse from the mother's drinking and verbal assaults also forced the child to turn elsewhere for affection and protection. The child would run outside and cry in agony or hide in a closet and withdraw into herself mentally. The withdrawal and crying process served to expand her latent psychic abilities, which in turn reinforced her perception of the Little People, the spirits who heard the child's crying and came to comfort and protect her.

At first the Little People appeared as what adults would consider imaginary playmates. However, Tela claimed that the Little People were not projections from the child's unconscious mind, but were in fact real psychic entities, who became constant companions of the child, especially during periods of torment, abuse, and neglect.

Tela held a meeting with the Little People during the healing ceremony and convinced them to relinquish their control over the child's mind and soul. She then entered the child's mind psychically, via telepathic communication, and convinced her that certain people could see and hear what she was really doing in "that other world." Tela gently (verbally, spiritually, and mentally) persuaded the little girl to speak, using the child's allies as part of the persuasion team. In other words, she persuaded the Little People to encourage the child to communicate with herself and with her mother.

The Little People told the child it was safe for her

to leave them and re-enter the physical world, with the understanding that she could always return to them if the situation ever became fearful. This negotiation between the shaman, the child's soul, and the invisible playmates proved to be successful, as the child cried, talked, and then timidly went over to her mother. Both mother and child were encouraged to talk to the Little People, thanking them for their assistance. Tela climaxed her ceremony with mother, child, spirits, and herself all singing together happily.

The mother confessed her neglect of the child. She apologized to the child and the spirits for the abuse and promised to seek professional psychotherapy. She also promised to spend more time with her child in cultural and traditional Native activities. On the third night of the healing, mother and child were purified together in a sacred sweat lodge ceremony.

Three years later the child was healthy, more intelligent than her peers in school, and had become very active in the local ceremonies. She claimed she still heard and saw her imaginary playmates, especially during dreams, times of ceremony, and in certain situations when she needed personal advice and guidance to deal with a problem. The mother quit drinking and partying and eventually remarried. It appears that the mother, stepfather and child are a close-knit and happy family.

Psychic phenomena, psychic symbols, religious convictions, and cultural concepts are not part of the Western biomedical approach, whereas the shamanistic approach includes a mixture of the psychological, behavioral, socio-cultural, physical, mythological, and spiritual (psychic phenomena).

The Native healer doctoring a White patient can sometimes be faced with the same problems encountered by the White doctor treating a Native. They have differences in beliefs and cultural heritage; both the White doctor's and the shaman's medical systems are culturally biased. What, then, makes Native healers so effective in the treatment of non-Native patients? The key is in the Native healer recognizing the possibility that non-Native patients may have preliterate or traditional beliefs too; that is, the patient may believe that his or her disease is the result of personal transgression ("I must have done something,") or malevolence ("Something or somebody must be doing this to me!"). The shaman attempts to grasp the patient's idea of the cause of the illness so that patient and healer can work closely together. Hence the healer inquires of both the Native and non-Native patient, "What kind of signs [omens] have you seen around your house?" or, "What kinds of dreams have you had lately?" The Western doctor, on the other hand, inquires "How do you feel?" The patient responds, "I feel as if my stomach is twisted up and full of snakes!" The White doctor authoritatively states, "Well, we'll take some X-rays and lab tests and find out what is really making you sick." The shaman would respond, "Well, we'll talk to those snakes and find out why they are tormenting you."

There may not be snakes in the patient's stomach in a physical sense, but they could be there in a psychic sense. Psychic phenomena normally do not show up on X-ray and lab test results, but they can be seen clairvoyantly. They can also be diagnosed and perhaps identified psychologically through dream interpretation. This is because the unconscious mind or soul communicates to the brain and the body through a complex system of symbols. These symbols are primal, natural, archetypal symbols. The shaman can "see" and understand such symbols, but typically White doctors function according to an entirely different set of symbols, which have been converted into a logical and limited left-brain system of language.

The conscious mind of the Western doctor may not be aware of these more primal symbols, but evidently the unconscious mind of the patient, Native or Western, and the psychic-oriented mind of the shaman are aware, and hence respond accordingly. In order to heal the patient, the source of "stress"—the symbol, the physical object, the form of power, and the fear associated with it—must be transformed or eradicated. It does not matter whether the therapist believes in the phenomenon, but he or she must recognize that the patient believes it. Simply changing the patient's belief system or forcing one's own belief system upon the patient will only serve to suppress or compound the problem.

The problem of not recognizing psychic phenomena is due to: 1) lack of awareness and special training on the part of the doctor or counselor; 2) a critical shortage of Western means to identify and handle such phenomena; and 3) inadequate preparation and training of professionals to deal with people who have culturally different beliefs, and to deal with the potential of psychic phenomena.

Assuming modern practitioners are willing to change their assumptions, they must find appropriate means or devices to discern phenomena that might be psychic in nature. Since average professionals cannot employ clairvoyance in diagnosing, perhaps they could hire a bonafide "psychic" as a consultant, one who has clearly demonstrated keen clairvoyant abilities and experience. The Tenrukyo Hospital in Japan and the London University in Great Britain are two sites at which efforts are being made to use such means to verify psychic phenomena in psychiatric situations. Perhaps American practitioners could learn from these recent experiments and develop new methods: conduct their own research, devise their own experiments, and make their own assumptions about the potential involvement of psychic phenomena as related to illness.

10 ▼ PLANT PEOPLE

▼   ▼   ▼   ▼   ▼   ▼

In the Beginning, when the Great Creator first made the world, He called together all the different spirits and asked them what they would like to be. Some wanted to be the Four Powers of the Universe, some wanted to be Lightning and Thunder, Wind, Rain, Snow, Earthquake. Some of the spirits said they would be oceans, mountains, rivers, and streams. The other spirits said they wanted to be the Plant people, Tree people, Animal people, Bird people, Fish people, Snake people, Bug people, Rock people, and Human people. In this way they would represent all those who walk, crawl, fly, and swim, seen and unseen. Together, they all made Creation.

By the use of ancient and esoteric creation stories our Elders teach us forms of knowledge which modern people are just now beginning to discover. In the above example we learn that all things have two sides, physical and spiritual, which serve to make the whole of any living thing. But we also learn that such things in creation are all interrelated and dependent upon each other for proper functioning and survival. And further, we learn that different forms have a different purpose and function in creation, and as part of creation they are all related to the Great Creator. Such philosophy, we may say, delves into metaphysics, but I would like to carry you a step further and sensitize you to the fact that the *meta* and the *physica* are interrelated and dependent upon each other. Logically we can try to separate the two and draw certain assumptions and conclusions, but in reality there is no separation. The physical and spiritual are One.

Such is the case in dealing with plants and people. We are all relations in this great Creation. You can spend a lifetime studying the botanical aspects of plants. You can become an expert in identifying the species, understanding each plant's individual chemistry, and learning how effectively to utilize its potential in healing in terms of a physical application. You can learn how to scientifically experiment with it in such a way as to develop a supposed better species, convert it into a domestic product, and even convert it into a hybrid species to make a product that is commercially more profitable. This may all work and even promote healing, in some people and in some cases.

However, a touch of spirit added somewhere in the process will make it far more powerful.

Our Elders teach us that there is more to things than meets the eye and mind. For example, suppose you and I are going for a walk in Nature. I pick up a stick, hand it to you, and ask, "What is this?" You respond by saying, "It is a piece of wood." After a few minutes, I remark, "No, it is a piece of a tree." Understand the difference? In our traditional Indian way we are taught to see the whole of each thing and attempt to understand its relationship to each part that makes the whole; how each part relates to other parts in Creation; how all parts serve to make the whole of Creation. In order to be more effective in the use of plants in healing, one must come to learn that a plant is a "whole" species. It is a living thing. It has a mind, body, and spirit. It can think, it has feelings, it can become sick or even die. It has four stages of evolutionary development, comparable to what human beings go through in a lifetime: it is born, it grows, it ages, and it dies; and most plants are born again.

Plants are "people" in the same way we are people. They are born into certain families; they have extended families, tribes, and nations; they also have friends and even enemies. Some work individually, but most prefer to work cooperatively. They have individual personalities which are influenced by physical chemistry and mental-spiritual thinking. A happy plant is a healthy plant; an unhappy plant is an unhealthy plant. A plant in its indigenous source of power is more potent and "powerful" than a domesticated species that has been cultivated. A natural plant gathered from its natural environment is more powerful in healing, especially if it is gathered in the right and proper way and at the right and proper time. Harvesting plants with prayer, ritual, and knowledge (communication formulas) will insure that the spirit of the plant stays with the body of the plant, and the plant will also be more effective in treatment for an illness.

Let me give you an example, a case study in the cultural context. A Native woman from northwestern California came to see me in a wheelchair. I could tell by the expression on her face that she was in severe pain. I didn't know at first exactly what was wrong, but I felt by the way my own bones and joints began to ache that she probably had some form of arthritis.

The woman was forty years old. She did not smoke and was divorced. She had been in a car accident ten years ago and had fractured several vertebrae and evidently ruptured a disc. According to her testimony the pain had progressed slowly over the years and came in cycles; there were high pain periods which were unbearable and moderate times where she could suppress the pain with aspirin. As the illness developed over the years she had no choice but to seek medical assistance, first her family physician and later a bone specialist. They both diagnosed her as having chronic osteo-arthritis in her spine, knees, neck, and joints. A series of medicines were used to alleviate the pain, such as motrin, cortisone, and phenylbutazolidin. Nothing seemed to work. At first she used crutches to help in her movement, but she had to periodically use the wheelchair to take the increasing weight gain off the injured and inflamed areas of her body. The illness was beginning to interfere seriously in her job, sex life, and personal life.

She asked if we would perform a traditional Native healing ceremony on her. I said we would need to pray on it first, talk to the Creator and spirits, and find out if we could help her. This is our way to find out if we are meant to take the case and to prepare for it, or if the ill person is meant to be healed. Sometimes we are told not to interfere because the person is meant to suffer for a violation or sin committed, or the spirits might tell us that we are not qualified to help this person, and then the patient is referred to a different medicine man or woman. The preparatory prayer time also provides us with an opportunity to study the omens, dreams, and aura of the patient.

I started my sacred fire and sweat lodge ceremony that night. During the ceremony and within the privacy of the lodge I talked to the Great Creator and asked for help. I asked the Creator and spirits for permission to accept the case, I asked that they show me the cause(s) of the woman's degenerative illness, and I asked that they show me what powers to use in healing. While in a meditation, I had a vision. I saw the woman's accident and the injury to her body. I also saw what was on her mind at that time, causing the stress and mental anguish. I saw the violations which the woman had committed.

During an altered state of consciousness the Bear talked to me and told me what medicine, songs, and healing to use. He said he would help me. The vision was vivid. I saw the Bear walking along the river singing. Then he sat down within a large patch of herbs and talked to them, picked an arm load, then handed the herbs to me. He said to use them in healing the woman, to boil them and have her drink the tea for four days straight and to bathe in it for four nights. He called it *ma-chan-ip,* which in the Yurok Indian language means wormwood.

The next morning I asked the patient to come to my house at sunset and we would begin a ceremony on her. She would have to stay with us for four days and nights. During this period my wife and I took turns singing, dancing, and doctoring her. I found the wormwood herbs exactly where the Bear had showed me in the vision, and at sunrise I gathered a batch with prayer and ritual; the instructions given in the sweat lodge were followed to the letter. By the fourth night the woman was completely healed and has not had any further disease, arthritis or otherwise. That was ten years ago and she is healthy, has remarried, and was promoted to a supervisor on her job.

Wormwood is a strong herbal healer. We have used it on numerous occasions with many different cases. We boiled it and bathed our children in it when they were infants for diaper rash, and it always cleared up. We have prescribed it for friends who had bad cases of jock itch or athlete's foot and they always cleared up. We have administered it to children and animals who had pin worms, scabies, or skin rashes. We have used it for bursitis, torn ligaments, sprains, other cases of arthritis, and even broken bones. We have even used it on serious head fractures and injuries; it was taken as a tea and the warm leaves wrapped around the injured spot like a poultice.

Some people claim wormwood was brought here by the Europeans, but the Elders say it has always been here. I have come to learn that there are several different species, some indigenous and some exotic. I have also learned that the concoction must be made in the proper dose and should not be consumed for more than a few days at a time because it can effect the liver.

Dreams and visions teach medicine people how to use plants and herbs, or they can learn by an apprenticeship. Some medicine people specialize in herbal doctoring. That is their main medicine and they do not delve into other kinds. These people fall into two categories: 1) those chosen by the Creator and spirits to use the power of herbs in healing; 2) those who buy the knowledge by studying under an older medicine man or woman. Native healers who become herbalists via dreams, visions, and the spiritual calling are always much stronger and more effective in healing than those who purchase the medicine. They use the spiritual power and medicine of plants in healing, while those in the second category rely solely on the chemical and physical properties. Sometimes this works and sometimes it does not. But if a plant or an animal that works with plants, such as a bear, talks to you in dreams and tells you it will be your teacher and ally, you really have the power.

I have met people who know a lot more about plants and herbs than I do. They can identify over 100 species, give the scientific names, and describe in detail how to use them. This is good survival knowledge and I respect them. But I will not use any plants unless the spirits have told me how to use them. I have been taught this by my Elders, by my spiritual allies, and by making mistakes.

Plants and herbs have a special place, purpose, and function upon this earth—to heal. In order to be effective in healing, we as humans must begin to recognize the fact that the whole plant(s) must be used in the healing process, its spiritual properties along with the physical properties. Plants are alive, and when gathered with prayer and hired to perform a job via ritual agreement and apology, they will provide added life energy to the ill person. The physical part of the plant works on the physical body of the patient, and the spiritual essence of the plant works on the spirit of the human. Thus plants and people have a harmonious relationship.

Plants are "people"; they can hear our thoughts, communicate, and respond. They communicate symbolically and telepathically, as in dreams and vision-seeking. In traditional Native doctoring the medicine people always make an effort to communicate with the plant before using it. They talk to it in the same way one would talk to a fellow being. They ask for its help, for permission to take its life and force, and they always offer payment of some kind (tobacco, money, beads, food, prayers of praise) in exchange for its life and service. They also address the plant's family, tribe, and relations in Nature, and ask for permission to remove the plant from its home since all things are related and each part is significant to the whole. In this way, they show respect to all living things. By demonstrating respect to that which God has created, they demonstrate respect to God. No man or woman can heal without the power and blessing of the Great Creator.

prayer formula

O Great Creator, I come before you in a humble way and ask for your help. I ask that you loan me your power in healing and your medicine from Creation. I come before you plant people with a good heart and ask for your assistance. I understand that you were put here on the Earth from the very Beginning of Time to help human beings. You are a healer. I am sorry that I have to take your life, but according to ancient custom and law, I offer you this tobacco and prayer as payment. I ask your family and all your relations in Nature for permission to take your life, and I offer them payment. I ask that your mind, body, and spirit doctor the mind, body, and spirit of the patient. I pray for your people, I give thanks to your people, and I wish you all long life and prosperity.

11 ▼ THE MEDICINE SWEAT

▼   ▼   ▼   ▼   ▼   ▼

*A LONG, LONG TIME AGO SICKNESS CAME TO THE FIRST
People. The world was in pain then—droughts, fires,
tornadoes, earthquakes, hurricanes, volcanic eruptions,
and floods raged across the earth. This was followed by
pestilence, poverty, sickness, fear, and disease. All things
began to die in great numbers.*

*It was decided that a council should be held to discuss
the problem. They came from every direction—the animal people, bird people, fish people, snake people, bug
people, plant people, tree people, rock people, and even
the human people.*

*For four days they fasted, prayed, meditated, and
sought visions and guidance, vowing to contribute their
knowledge, power, and medicine to help in some way.*

Eagle came in on a gust of wind from the north and said, "I have brought the first power of creation."

Flickerbird came in from the east and said, "I have brought fire, the second power of creation, for a sacred ceremony." And she flicked red sparks from her tail feathers into the center of the council meeting.

"Wait," said a green cedar tree, coming in from the south, "my relations and I have brought food for the sacred fire. Here, take some of my dry branches and tobacco from my little plant sister here with me."

In time the fire began to grow. It danced with the wind while the people sang. But soon it got too strong and the people became concerned.

Raven came flying in from the west. He was carrying a water-tight willow root basket. "Here," he said, "I have brought water and rocks. Perhaps we can encircle the fire and use the water to keep it under control."

Raven tried to build a small wall around the fire with rocks. It was contained but so hot it burned him completely black. He tripped trying to get away from the flames, knocking over the basket, and caused water to splash on the sacred fire. It began to steam all over.

Raven squawked for help and could no longer sing. "Quick," said Grizzlybear, "cover him with your hides." So Elk, Deer, and other large animals donated their skins as a protective covering. The people were so happy they started singing and dancing again. In this way they gave Raven community support with his problem.

When it was all over Raven was sweating. The austerity and suffering gave him a vision. "This is what we *shall use to save ourselves," he said. "The Great Spirit told me we should call this a sweat lodge, and it will be sacred to all the people." That is how Raven became a great doctor, but he is no longer a good singer.*

symbolic and conceptual description

An elderly holy man told me this creation story when I was being trained to become a doctor for our people. Like Raven, I too had to sweat, suffer, and sacrifice in order to qualify for the vision and powers to heal. And I had to have community support in order to become a servant, as did Raven.

As already mentioned, I was taught and trained in the ancient and esoteric art of medicine making by sixteen elderly ceremonial leaders and healers from different tribes, who were my mentors. The tribal myths were my scriptures and prayer formulas. Nature was my university, laboratory, and internship residency. And the sacred sweat lodge became my tool for self-discovery, apprenticeship, healing, and transpersonal development.

Sweat lodges used by tribes across the continent had a similar function: the sacred structure was a form of mini-church where individuals and small groups could talk to their Creator, their spirit guides, powers, soul, or each other about personal problems and needs. It was a place where one could figure out problems by seeking visions, using creative dreaming and imagination, or psychic guidance. The solution might come in the form of a myth, vivid dream, vision, special voice, or supernatural aid. Sometimes the answer was very clear, and other times it was vague, requiring more abstract thinking, concentration, and meditation.

The sweat lodge had additional applications. Some tribes utilized it in preparation for sports and games, perhaps similar to what is now called autogenic training. It was used in preparation for war when men attempted to make "protective medicine." Those who returned from war as survivors were purified in the sweat lodge to cleanse their soul of atrocities, repair injuries, remove potential mental flashbacks, and to protect themselves from tormenting "ghosts." The sweat lodge is still used today by some families to purify themselves after attending a burial ceremony or funeral. In these ways it served as a spiritual tool and a form of dealing with stress.

There are many different kinds of sweat lodge ceremonies, each requiring a special style, special knowledge, mode of operation, medicines, prayers, leaders, and paraphernalia. I usually advise neophytes to stay with the basics and just use water for steam, a pinch of pipe tobacco for an invocation, and a bit of cedar to purify the lodge and keep away the negative forces. I have been in hundreds of sweat lodge ceremonies and found no two were ever alike, whether conducted by myself or some other leader. I have sweated in both the Native American style of sweat lodges and the various kinds of Whiteman's/European style sweat houses. I have sweated with Sioux Sun Dancers who used a hundred rocks in one ceremony and in a medicine sweat where only one rock was used. The medicine sweat was conducted by a woman, my wife, Tela Starhawk, and it was the hottest and most powerful experience I have encountered yet. I have had sweats in clear weather, pouring rain, snow, ice, fog, high winds, droughts, and even during several earthquakes. I have experienced sweats in the early morning, at noon, after sunset, all night long, and even during specific star, moon, or planetary alignments. I was even fortunate to experience several ceremonies during both solar and lunar eclipses. In all these experiences I came to learn that the sweat lodge is, indeed, a sacred ceremony. It must be treated with respect, accountability, and according to the natural and aboriginal laws.

Some Native people conduct "mixed sweats" and others do not. In fact, in most tribes the women did not originally sweat with the men unless they were being doctored, past menopause, or training to be medicine women. In lieu of the sweat lodge they used the moontime ceremony held in a structure similar to the sweat lodge but more like a wickiup, called a moonlodge, moontipi, or menses hut. Today, however, certain Native women leaders and Elders feel that the sweat lodge ceremony is needed, in addition to the moontime ceremony, in order to purge themselves of all the poisons, pollutants, and illnesses created by Western civilization. But, again, pregnant women and menstruants are asked not to participate in the sweat lodge for health reasons.

The four powers of "Creation" serve as the main source of healing and medicine for the sweat lodge. This medicine is reflected in the construction and application of the lodge, and it is utilized in the symbolic, spiritual, physical, and mental dynamics of the sweat lodge experience. The four powers, four elements, four colors, and four forces are eternal and infinite; they serve to form what Jung called a universal archetype and "quaternity," while the lodge itself is like a mandala.

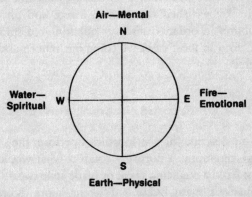

The sweat lodge is circular; hence, we are cautioned to think positive thoughts and make good prayers for the Great Creator, the Mother Earth, each other, ourselves, or for a specific patient. It is not a place to make curses, bad wishes, or bad prayers because the power of the circle always returns to its original starting point. So part of the sweat lodge ceremony involves discipline and learning. We discipline our thoughts and actions and we learn how to channel certain energies in a positive, creative, and appropriate manner.

We prefer to go into the sacred sweat lodge naked, stripped of all our clothes, symbols, badges of education and status, wealth, camouflages, or other coverings which feed the human ego. We go naked as a newborn into the womb of our Mother Earth; humble, pure, innocent, and prepared for nurturing. We try to strip ourselves of all the human qualities, desires, and characteristics in order to become more spirit-like; we shed our human image and physical attributes in order to discover our soul and spiritual side. And in most cases we come out reborn and re-created.

construction and method

Let me describe the way in which I perform the sweat lodge ceremony. I normally conduct what would be considered a medicine sweat or turtle style sweat. The shamanistic sweat lodge is different, more rigorous, more intense, and sometimes requires toughening up in order to deal with the austerity. I have found the medicine sweat to be the most effective, although it is criticized by some of my peers as not being elaborate enough. I appreciate elaboration and understand the need for specific procedures, objects, colors, and paraphernalia in such ceremonies, but my emphasis is on quality, not quantity. I do not rely upon a larger number of rocks to make it hotter or more powerful.

My objective is to use the sacred sweat lodge for doctoring, healing, spiritual development, vision seeking, therapy, and holistic health. Although I know how to conduct sweat lodges in different styles and ways I prefer the medicine approach. My ceremony and lodge is simple and small but highly effective.

If I need to start out from scratch I follow one procedure; if the lodge is already constructed I use somewhat of a different procedure. Here is the process for starting from scratch.

First I walk around the land, pray and ask the Mother Earth and my relations in Nature for their permission to build a sacred sweat lodge in their territory. I explain who I am, where I come from, what the sweat lodge will be used for, and I promise to be respectful in their home. I offer them tobacco by smoking my pipe and sprinkling the leaves on the ground. I scout for a safe, level, and private space, and I try to feel a "node" or a power point where the four cardinal directions of the universe crisscross. I feel it intuitively or sometimes "see" the blue energy converging upon the ground. You can also find a node by using a "witching device" or dowsing rod such as metal hangers or willow branches.

I prefer the lodge to be located near a creek, stream, lake, or pond, but if needed I will add a large tank or tub and water hose for bathing after the sweat. Sometimes I ask the spirits to show me a sign or omen as to where to put the lodge. For example, I was asked to build a new camp sweat lodge for Rolling Thunder out in Nevada several years ago. I spent some time surveying the environment, prayed, and asked for a sign. A flickerbird flew in from the east, sat upon a particular spot, whistled, then danced. I knew then without a doubt where to build the lodge.

Next I thank the spirits in Nature, walk over to the node, sit upon the ground facing north, pray, and begin to address the four sacred directions and powers of the universe. I ask each to lend us its power and to bless the spot and make it holy ground in keeping with the ancient creation story and formula. I first start with the Air in the north, then rotate to the east (Fire), south (Earth), and finally the west (Water). I sit upon the ground meditating and giving thanks, trying to merge my consciousness with the great cosmic consciousness and to feel the power of the earth energy merge with my own vibratory level. In this way I establish a connection with the Mother Earth and create my own "center of the world." I have taught the same procedure to my White brothers who wanted to build a Finnish style steam sauna, and they found it works for their system too.

Next, I take out two sticks and some string and draw a circle sunwise, approximately four feet from the center of the node. I make a smaller circle for the rock hole, get a shovel, offer tobacco at the earth node, and apologize for breaking its skin. Then I dig a small hole approximately a foot and a half deep and a foot in diameter. I place the dirt outside the circle, facing east, for the altar.

The second step involves gathering the willows. Each part of gathering and constructing the sacred sweat lodge must be prayed on according to the law of reciprocity. (I usually fast during the construction of my sweat lodges and even abstain from water.) In order to carry the life force, the spirit and energy of the tree as a medicine into the sweat lodge, we must make a prayer offering and ask its permission to share its life and body. So we walk up to the tree people and repeat an ancient prayer formula for this purpose, which basically states that the willow tree is special because it represents the four seasons of nature, the four powers of the universe, the four stages of humankind, and because its life is cyclic. We offer it tobacco, herbs, money, or beads as payment for taking its life. Then we cut carefully. All smaller limbs are replanted in the ground with a special wish that they will grow and prosper. Willow trees are normally found along creeks, streams, and rivers. The tall, lean saplings are best.

The willows are brought back to the site of the sweat lodge and the bark peeled off. I usually gather sixteen or twenty saplings, approximately one to two inches thick. The long strips of bark can be used for natural string to tie the structure (some people prefer to use modern twine), or they can be saved as headache medicine.

Four small holes approximately three inches deep are poked into the ground with a tire iron or steel bar, spaced directly across from each other on the circular line; they should be facing north and south, then east and west. The stout end of the sapling is sharpened to a point and placed firmly in the hole and packed tightly. I then stand in the middle and bend the top ends toward each other, slowly so they will not work loose and fly up in my face. I bend them until they are about chest high and tie them. I proceed to each set until a structure and frame has been shaped (see illustration). By the time all eight saplings are secured at the crossing joints, I can crawl under the frame and begin the side lacing. I usually interweave two rolls around the side to form a more solid hull. Lastly, I make a horseshoe-shaped sapling for the door and place it in the front entrance facing east. It is always easier if two people participate in the construction of the lodge.

Next come the hides, canvas, old rugs, or tarps. I always smudge the material to remove potential contamination and negative energy, then carefully spread and shape it over the structure. My sweat lodge is turtle shaped, rather small, and can accommodate about seven people. My friend Archie Fire Lamedeer, a Sioux medicine man, makes his lodge big and round, to hold over sixteen people. But I am a short man in comparison to Archie, who is six foot four inches tall and large in build. So one may gauge the size of the lodge according to the size of the leader and participants. I normally use four to seven rocks per ceremony, while Archie typically uses sixteen to forty, depending on the kind of medicine being made. As you can see, lodges vary in size and in the way they are used.

Once the sweat lodge is completed I begin work on the sacred fire pit for the rocks. I count ten feet east from the door, make a line, walk seven feet across, and make another line. I find the center point, pull out my sticks and string, and make a large circle in a clockwise direction. I offer tobacco to the earth, apologize for hurting it and any bug people, then proceed to dig a hole for the pit, approximately a foot deep. The dirt is used to form a wall.

Now we are ready for the rocks. There are several kinds that are good for sweating, but all of them should be hard, gathered from a good, clean place in Nature, and gathered by prayer. Sandstone bursts and should be avoided. The favorite choices are lava rocks, blue river rocks, and high mountain rocks with ore instead of quartz.

Rocks are alive; they have special power, and must be treated with respect at all times. Therefore I sit upon the ground in front of the "family" and explain why I need their help. I offer tobacco (and sometimes money) as payment and apologize to the family for removing them from their home. I select only those I "feel" are willing to sacrifice themselves as medicine for the ceremony. Sometimes, if we listen carefully, we can "hear" them sing and talk to us in response; in other situations I feel the life of the rock by caressing it and connecting with its energy. A cold, withdrawn rock does not want to be bothered; a warm, vibrating rock is eager to be used. Larger rocks are placed around the sacred fire pit and smaller ones, softball to soccer ball size, are heated for the ceremony. (In the Finnish style steam sauna one must choose much smaller rocks, from the size of the human fist to that of a baseball.)

I choose only rocks which my spirit guides tell me to use, and only the number they dictate to apply in the ceremony. I am a "spiritual" doctor, which means I let the spirits conduct the ceremony instead of trying to conduct it myself. If they want it hot, it will be hot; if they do not want it hot, it will not get hot no matter how many rocks I use.

Next comes the wood, which is a very important ingredient for any kind of sweat lodge. Some people have their wood cut, split, stacked, and preseasoned before the ceremonies. Sometimes we need to gather it on the same day. It is always best if the wood is gathered in a "ceremonial way" by prayer. Trees are sacred; they too have power and a special life force to contribute as medicine, and they are very sensitive. So we make prayers to the tree people and all those who share their abode, asking for their assistance. We apologize to them for taking their life.

Now I realize that all of this may sound silly to the typical logical Westerner, but our Native people have always been more intuitive and holistic in their approach to gathering natural resources. We believe that each piece, part, or element contributes a special life force and spirit to the ceremony, that all things are alive and possess a spirit, and everything in nature is a form of medicine if one knows how to recognize and use it. Each rock, for example, has its own form of communication and vibratory level which affects its energy pattern and frequency; hence it is alive. For this reason I never use rocks in my ceremony that have been used in a previous ceremony; such rocks are indeed dead because their life force has been sapped, channeled into the circle of power, and transmitted into the participants. Trees, too, are not just dead wood but energy forces combined with the rocks and natural elements to create a special kind of physical and spiritual energy. Credence is lent to our Native perspective by a scientific study (Tompkin and Bird, 1972) that shows that plants talk and respond to human communication; and studies at Harvard concluded that trees also talk to each other.

An alchemy of tree knowledge is an important ingredient for the medicine-making part of the sweat lodge ceremony. For example, the higher up one goes to gather the wood, the stronger the power will be in the ceremony. Live wood has more force and power than seasoned wood gathered commercially and without ceremony; and the way in which the wood is mixed for the ceremony affects the temperature of the fire and rocks. When possible, I like to combine four different kinds of wood in my ceremony: green soft, green dry, hard dry, and hard green wood. The age, texture, species, location, and chemical composition of the trees serve to make certain recipes for healing certain kinds of illnesses. Since each tree is alive it can contribute a different kind of energy to the mixture, causing a weak force, strong force, fast force, or slow force. My favorites include a combination of cedar with oak or madrone, or fir and locust, depending upon the environment and location. Of course, there may be times when a person must use whatever is available, for instance when sweats are conducted in prisons or in the Finnish style steam sauna. Even then, however, I always take the time to bless and give thanks to the wood by blessing and smudging it with cedar or sage smoke.

the fire

Finally, I begin construction of the sacred fire. At this point I usually light my pipe, pray to the Great Creator and four sacred directions, and ask for their assistance and powers. If it is raining I ask that the sky be opened and made temporarily clear. If it is too windy, posing a fire hazard, I ask for calmness and cooperation of the wind and fire. If there is no wind, I request breath to start the sacred fire. I state the reason why I am conducting a sweat lodge ceremony, I name the people who will be involved, and I state the need for certain kinds of healing. Then I pick out four blocks of wood to create a square altar, place rocks upon the altar, smudge all the rocks, and continue to stack the wood in a circular fashion, starting with the dry soft that leads into the outer layers of dry and green hardwood. I sing sweat lodge songs, calling in different spirits for protection, support, and power assistance. But I always leave an opening for the "eastern door" which is used to attract light, force, and energy from the Grandfather Sun, and to light the fire ceremony. This energy from the Sun follows a set pattern; it goes into the fire pit, then into the front door at the sweat lodge, then into the center hole of the lodge, where the rocks will eventually be placed after heating. From the macrocosm to the microcosm. From the giant solar system of which we are all a part, to our individual selves which in reality are also a form of solar system.

Some finishing touches should be mentioned here. I always place cedar, pepperwood leaves, or sage upon my altar prior to lighting the fire, and I ask for protection. This medicine serves to keep away the bad spirits and powers and attract only the good spirits. And I usually smudge the inside of the sweat lodge with sage or sweetgrass, although the floor of the lodge has already been lined with Douglas fir boughs, cedar boughs, or mugwort.

In order to focus on the ritualistic ingredients of the ceremony I need an assistant, and I choose someone to be fire keeper. This is an honorable position and requires dedication, willingness to follow orders, and a sincere heart to handle the responsibilities associated with the duty. The fire keeper must make sure that the fire is properly fed and not let it get out of hand. This person is responsible for taking the rocks out of the fire, transferring them to the sweat lodge, and handing the leader the power objects and medicines needed in the ceremony. As a result, the fire keeper either comes into the lodge last, or on certain occasions must forfeit the opportunity to sweat while performing additional duties such as caring for the sick patient who might leave the lodge early.

While the fire is being tended by the fire keeper, I continue to pray and sing. By this time I have provided an orientation. I reserve some time to speak in privacy with those who need counseling, and I encourage the participants to engage in preparatory sweat lodge songs. These are normally sung in sets of four. In essence they are ancient hymns and prayer formulas, not simply chants. I ask the participants to abstain from drugs, sex, alcohol, and sometimes coffee for one to four days prior to the ceremony, during the ceremony, and for another one to three days after the ceremony, and I am under the same restrictions. On occasion I ask the patient and/or participants to fast and refrain from food and water from one to four days. We do this, for example, in preparation for the spring equinox, the summer solstice, the fall equinox, and winter solstice ceremonies. By allowing a period of being clean we are also allowing ourselves an opportunity to be purified and to receive visions, and time for the medicine to work. Also fasting and staying clean makes the power and ceremony stronger.

I rarely sweat with women unless they are being doctored or training to be medicine women; and I never sweat with women on their menses. Hence I seldom conduct mixed sweats. Women are accommodated in the sweat lodge ceremony by my wife, so in this way I can follow my own religious beliefs and laws and not be blamed for discrimination.

It usually takes about two hours for the wood pile to burn down and the rocks to get hot and ready. In the meantime I prepare water for the bathing tank and for the sweat lodge water bucket. I pray to the water in a certain way, asking its spirit and energy to help us. I ask that it purify our mind, body, soul, and I ask it to share with us strength, protection, long life, and good health. Whatever time is left after praying, singing, counseling, and checking the fire keeper's performance is spent preparing myself psychically to conduct the ceremony. I meditate, seek guidance from my spirits, and let the spiritual power flow through me so I can channel it to the participants.

the sweat

Now we are ready to sweat. I ask everyone to take a quick urine break, shed their clothes, put personal items on the altar to be blessed, and form a line to enter the lodge. I also advise all participants to remove glasses and jewelry so they will not get burned. As the leader, I crawl in first, followed by the patient, and then the next in line. I crawl in on my hands and knees like a bear, and humble myself before the spirits as we all enter into the womb of our Mother Earth. I take my "medicine bundle," herbs, and power objects with me and at the doorway ask, "All my relations please accept me into the sacred circle of life."

The participants follow, repeating the same prayer until each is seated within a circle, facing the center hole where the rocks will be placed.

As each rock is brought in it is arranged to represent the four sacred directions: mental (N), emotional (E), physical (S), and spiritual (W). The remaining rocks represent our ancestors, Elders, women, and children, and special prayers are made for them on these rocks. The fire keeper enters last and the flap is closed.

I invoke the Great Creator, the Mother Earth, the four sacred directions, the spirits, and all our relations in Nature. I also pray to the different power places where I have trained, the mountains I am connected to, and the different spirits I work with in ceremony and healing. We pray and give thanks to the Great Creator; we pray for the Elders, the women and children, and for the brothers and sisters who are in prison. We pray for our families, friends, each other, and ourselves. We confess our sins and violations we have made against Nature, the Creator's laws, or for any harm we have done to other human beings; we ask to be forgiven for harming, hurting, insulting, or doing injury to any living creature in Nature, seen or unseen.

Participants are encouraged to state their problem or illness and ask for healing. Sometimes this leads to confessing violation of a natural, moral, spiritual, or manmade law. Confessing is good for the soul, and it serves as a catharsis in our form of Native psychotherapy. Inside the sacred sweat lodge people can confess in privacy and in group confidentiality while the sweats and medicines purify them. It also serves to rid the psyche of deep-seated guilt or shame.

The songs we use in the sweat lodge are culturally specific and hence vary from tribe to tribe. I usually have the participants sing a welcoming song to the newcomers, and we sing specific sweat lodge songs. I always sing a variety of healing songs, some ancient and willed to me by the Elders, and some I have received from the Creator and spirits during different vision quests.

As I pour water upon the rocks I pray for the participants and fan them with an eagle wing. In some situations I might make up an herbal tea, pour it on the rocks, and have the patients drink it for healing and purging. If a person is in pain or injured I go into a trance and let certain doctor spirits work through me. I often use my hands to pull the sickness out and throw it into the rocks where the spirits grab it and carry it deep down into the center of the earth. If patients have to vomit to release pain, sickness, fear, stress, anxiety, or depression, they are advised to do it into the fir boughs behind them and not into the rocks. Whatever negative energy, toxins, or illness we may have is drained through the earthfloor and destroyed by the spirits so it cannot return.

We might stay in the lodge only fifteen minutes or until daybreak. When the spirits tell me it is time to get out, we get out. Sometimes we might take a break, refresh ourselves, and go back in for additional praying, vision-seeking, healing, discussion, or guidance. Anyone who wants can leave without ridicule after the invocation by simply calling out, "All my relations." I do not like macho power trips in the sweat lodge ceremony. I recognize that each person's tolerance level is different, so anyone who finds it too hot or powerful can leave gracefully and with respect, including me! I don't appreciate sweat lodge ceremonies that are conducted with power games where people try to see who is the toughest, the strongest, or who has the most power. I feel that this kind of attitude is wrong for a spiritual ceremony and hence do not allow it. My sweats are simple, designed for healing, and require very little elaboration, although I respect those that are different.

bathing

We come out of the lodge and jump into the creek or water tank. As we bathe we pray to the spirit of the water and ask for strength, protection, long life, and good health; and we thank the water for its cleansing. Then we dry off, sit around the fire, and reflect on our experience, letting the medicines slowly continue working on us. If needed we talk about certain kinds of phenomena we may have seen or experienced in the sweat and try to understand it. All the sickness, stress, problems, and negative energy is left behind in the sweat lodge where it will be absorbed into the holy circle and diffused. Therefore, I usually remove the tarp the next day and let the elements purify the lodge before using it again.

a sauna sweat lodge

I have used basically the same approach in the Whiteman's Finnish style steam sauna, which uses a wood heater. The sauna style can be effective if it is constructed and applied in a good spiritual way. The four powers, four elements, four sacred directions are also in the sauna type sweat house, and it too can be used for healing, therapy, holistic health, and spiritual development. Tobacco ties can be made with special prayers and placed in the four corners and cedar burned. Sweat lodge prayers and procedures can be used, and herbal medicines can be employed effectively with various power objects. If the steam type sauna is treated as a sacred dwelling, it will attract good spirits and provide a healing experience.

In some ways the square Whiteman's style might be more appropriate to use in dealing with modern sicknesses because it can be constructed more readily in the city environment, and it requires less wood. Whatever style a person chooses to construct and apply, however, should be treated with respect, as a sacred ceremony, and as professional and spiritual medicine that requires a sense of responsibility. Both the circle and the square are what Jung called universal archetypes and have power. Symbols are effective tools in transpersonal development and therapy.

an ancient medicine for modern
sickness

I believe the sacred sweat lodge, round or square, ancient or modern, can be used as a means to doctor people, in the way I have been doctoring, for diseases such as arthritis, cancer, leukemia, Hodgkins disease, influenza, mental illness, or against stress and sorcery. It can be used for rites of passage to provide therapy for adolescents, during life crisis stages, for marriage and family counseling, and for stress management. When I was in college, I went into the sweat at the end of each quarter to purify my mind, body, and soul and relieve stress. I have used the sacred sweat lodge to help veterans overcome flashbacks, to doctor people tormented by ghosts and spirits, and those with nightmares. I have used the sweat lodge cere-mony to marry people, to celebrate the birth of a newborn, and as a cleansing after funerals. And I firmly believe that the sweat lodge can prove to be one of the most valuable medicines in the treatment of alcohol and drug abuse, especially for our Native American people. It might be an ancient medicine but it has the potential to deal effectively with a wide range of modern illnesses.

sweat lodge prayer

Great Creator, we come before you in a humble manner and ask for your help. We offer these herbs and pray. To the four sacred directions and powers of the Universe we pray: to the spirits of the air in the north, to the spirits of the fire in the east, to the spirits of the earth in the south, and to the spirits of the water in the west.

We pray and give thanks to you, O Great Spirit. We pray and give thanks to the Grandfather Sun, the Grandmother Moon, to the Mother Earth, and all our relations in Nature. We thank you for your power, energy, gifts, and resources, because without you we would not be able to live and survive. We ask that you forgive us if we have ever harmed or hurt you. We pray, offer this tobacco and herbs, and ask that you doctor us, heal us, purify us, and protect us. We pray for our Elders, women, children, and fellow human beings. We ask for peace, harmony, and healing worldwide.

12 ▼ NATIVE PRACTICES FOR HEALING YOURSELF

▼   ▼   ▼   ▼   ▼   ▼

THERE ARE SOME PRACTICES THAT CONTEMPORARY WESTerners can learn from the Native healer for self-healing. For example, you can teach yourself to use your dreams as a learning tool. Before you go to bed at night do some self-talking and visualization. Talk to your mind and soul. Tell your mind that you want to see your dreams clearly, but you do not want to see any of the trivial, useless dreams. Tell your mind that you want to remember important dreams and to wake you up whenever you feel you are in danger. This takes practice and discipline. The Elders taught me to create a ritual for it. I burn cedar, medicine roots, or smoke my sacred pipe and pray to the Great Creator and good powers just before going to sleep. During the prayer I state my name, race, tribe, and a clear request. I say something like this:

> "O Great Creator and the good doctor spirits. I offer you this tobacco and sacred cedar. I ask for your help. I want to learn how to develop and use my dreams, to remember my dreams, and to learn from my dreams. I ask that the spirit of the cedar and good powers protect me while I experiment with this dreaming power. I ask that my soul be my teacher and protector. I ask that I be given a dream ally who will serve as my teacher, adviser, and guardian. I ask that you protect me from all bad thoughts, powers, and entities. Teach me how to creatively develop my dreams, to use dreams to answer certain questions, to resolve problems in my life, or to decipher dreams that I don't understand."

Recording dreams is a good habit to develop. Don't be disappointed if you don't dream every night or if you can't remember every dream. Some dreams are just not meant to be remembered or recorded. At first you might have to put a notebook and pencil next to your bed as a means to record the dreams immediately when you wake up. When I first started there were times that I had to use a tape recorder for some dreams that came from the "deep sleep realm" and caused me to wake up groggy. Your retention ability will get better with practice. Eventually, through discipline and training you will automatically or subconsciously program your mind to remember and retain dreams that are significant.

Another good habit to develop is analyzing dreams at breakfast time. Share your dreams confidentially with your spouse and children. Get in the habit of discussing dreams and analyzing each other's dreams at a certain time each day or several times a week. The more you think about dreams, the more you talk about them, and the more you analyze them, the better you will become at developing the power of dreaming.

Native style meditation is another practice Westerners can use. I built an altar in one of my spare rooms and set up my Native religious items and power objects to symbolically and spiritually serve as spirit allies. I sit facing east, smudge myself with cedar, offer tobacco to the four sacred directions. Some people use an abalone shell for smudging, but I prefer to use an old grinding rock.

I meditate by using breathing exercises and visualization. I light a white candle to represent the sacred fires I have used in our ceremonies and the prayer pits and altars we build while on a vision quest on the mountain top. I focus my attention on the dancing flame, sing a prayer song, take four deep breaths that are exhaled slowly as I count backward from seven to one. I try to visualize a waterfall, a mountain lake, a river, or a very peaceful place in Nature I have visited.

I try to see and relive that previous experience in my mind, smelling the trees and plants, feeling the warm breeze, hearing the hypnotic sound of the water. I keep telling myself that I will become totally relaxed, and I try to let the relaxation slowly move from the top of my head all the way down to my toes.

Then I visualize the bright, warm power of the Grandfather Sun slowly cleansing and recharging each of my psychic centers that are connected to the major glands in my endocrine system. Sometimes I visualize a waterfall doing the cleansing. While meditating I repeat an affirmation: "I will be strong, I will be healthy, I will be happy, I will be protected, I will have long life." Then I hum "I will be one with the Sun" four times. When I do this I can actually feel my vibratory level rising and all the tension, anger, and frustration leaving my mind, body, and soul. Sometimes I see an eagle come soaring in and try to merge my consciousness with his and fly through the sky, so relaxed, peaceful, and happy.

At the end of my ritual I use a special quartz crystal to recharge each of my psychic centers. I place the crystal on each gland until I can feel the warm healing power re-energizing the vital spiritual point. Then it bursts outward throughout my entire body with a re-newed life force. At the end of my twenty-minute meditation and ritual, I clean up my sacred crystal by washing it in running water. The crystal must be cleaned after each use because it pulls negative energy out of our bodies, and this must be transferred back to the earth or we will absorb it the next time we use the crystal.

If you don't know any Native songs, you can use specially designed, sound-oriented meditation tapes; such tapes use flutes, drums, sounds of Nature such as the ocean, wind, etc. On warm, sunny days I will do my meditation outside in a quiet park or on the outskirts of the city. If I am too uptight, I will drink a tea made from peppermint or camomile to help me relax.

Along with these alternatives however, I seriously believe most people need vitamin supplements and guidance. The vitamins don't have to be taken every day, only every other day; and you have to be careful not to overdose on vitamins A and D. I strongly suggest the use of natural foods, a diet high in vegetables and fruits and low in fats, salts, and cholesterol, along with vitamin supplements since the traditional Native foods are not available to everyone.

Lastly, I believe that regular use of the sacred sweat lodge ceremony will help to purge our systems of the toxins and negative energy we accumulate daily from Western civilization and pollution. As stated earlier, the sweat lodge can be used for stress management, as a means to deal with alcohol and substance abuse, and for spiritual growth, development, and healing. In the previous chapter I explained how to do a sweat. Here is another ritual and natural power you can use for good health.

To tap into the power of the Sun, you must get up just before sunrise, go out and make prayers, sing and dance, and give thanks to the Grandfather Sun. Give thanks for meeting the new day with a new life. Let that power and energy flow into you.

Take a glass of water with you. Talk and pray to it, to the spirit of the water as well as to the Grandfather Sun. If you are sick, hurt, or having bad luck, or if you have been damaged in any way, ask the Grandfather Sun to shine his strong healing power, beauty, and light into that water. After you have prayed for your family and yourself, drink that water. It will doctor you, heal you, and strengthen you. Why? Because all things in the Universe must have light. Our own inner soul, our inner being, also needs light because it too is a source of power. Our soul is just like the Sun. We are miniature Universes. Unfortunately, some of us are dim or our light has gone out. Thus the Sun can be used to recharge us. It is a profound source of power; without the Sun, nothing can live. And so it is with our own soul. In order to develop the power of love or any other power, we must first learn to light up our soul with the original power of creation, the universal Light.

The most important method and ceremony for spiritual development is the vision quest or power quest. All races of human beings were given this knowledge in the Beginning and we should relearn how to use it today.

The elderly people taught me different kinds of power acquisitions, where to go for it, what to say, and how to do it. I will share some of this, so when you decide you are ready to go on a power quest or vision quest you will now know what to do. Take tobacco, whether you smoke it or not, because that is what the spirits in this part of the world like, though oats and corn meal are acceptable substitutes. Some might prefer corn meal or corn blossoms, but the majority like tobacco. Offer that tobacco to the Creator and the spirit of that power spot. After you have started to fast, don't drink water. You never drink water when you are on a power quest because it will break your power and your medicine and flush the new power out of you. You can take a little herbal juice or fruit juice, or you can drink the liquid from some ground-up corn or a can of corn to keep you going.

When you get to the power spot, inside of a redwood tree, next to a waterfall, on a high mountain, in the middle of the desert, or in a cave, build a little fire and offer tobacco to the Great Creator, then to the spirits of the east, the south, the west, and the north. Introduce yourself: "Great Creator, Mother Earth, and all the Good Spirits and all my relations in Nature, my name is _____, I come from _____, my race is _____, my nationality is _____, and this is why I am here _____. According to ancient custom and law, I feed you tobacco" [sprinkle tobacco in the fire; if you don't have a fire, put it in the palm of your hand and blow it to the east]. After this you state very clearly why you want this power and what you intend to do with it. You state that if this power is loaned to you, it will not be permanent. It is only loaned because if you do not handle it in a right and proper way, it will kick back on you or be taken away. So you promise you will handle it in a right, proper, and good way.

Then make your prayer and keep it short and right to the point. Stay awake for as long as you can and watch, listen, and observe. (You should leave the power spot when you need to.)

Whatever comes in physically to greet you or makes contact with you is a source of power. Whatever you dream is also a source of power, unless it is just trivial. It is up to you if you want to stay there one day and night or four days and nights. Four days and nights of fasting for a power quest in most cases is sufficient, especially if you purify yourself as part of the preparation.

When you come down off the mountain or out of the wilderness or cave, you must bathe again. If you had a dream or a vision, you must record it and study it. If you don't understand it, take it to a spiritual adviser, a medicine man or woman or even a good psychic you trust. Do not tell everybody about what you saw and heard or what you got in the dream or vision for at least a year, or you will lose it. It takes time for the power to be absorbed into your being.

Once you are back it is good to go into the sweat house again and purify yourself. Try and stay away from other people for at least three or four more days and nights. You want to be pure and have your mind focused and everything straight before you go to that power place, and you want to stay clean and pure with good thoughts while you are there. When you come down you want to stay clean for another few days and nights to let the power settle into you. If you eat in a restaurant or get drunk and party or make love or eat with people who may have negative energy in them, it will break your power and your medicine. You need time to cook it, as we say, to have it become one with you, and be absorbed.

It also takes a long time to study the power. Don't go up there and ask for everything in the world; be humble about it. Maybe ask for just one thing. It is better to know the correct use of just one kind of medicine, one kind of herb, one kind of plant, one kind of rock, one kind of song, one kind of dream, or one kind of power than to try and get more power and become careless.

I have shared a number of shamanistic practices present-day people can use for spiritual development and growth without violating Native religion. The vision quest, the sweat lodge, and some kind of ritual associated with menses have been used by all cultures at one time. A survey of world-wide literature also indicates that most societies originally used dream development and therapy, and some Western groups still practice the ancient art of dreaming for spirituality. So the shamanistic information I have tried to share in this book is not just lessons about my Native religious beliefs, customs, and esoteric teachings; it is a reinforcement and elaboration of ancient knowledge with the hope of encouraging all of us toward a more spiritual life. That is in essence what our Native people have always tried to do for our people—and we are all the Great Creator's people and people of the earth. Perhaps now we can begin to share, to learn, to grow, and to evolve spiritually together as our ancient Native American prophecies predicted would occur.

13 ▼ THE NATIVE HEALER IN
TODAY'S SOCIETY

▼   ▼   ▼   ▼   ▼   ▼

THERE IS A LOT WE CAN LEARN FROM THE NATIVE spirituality and what it takes to become a medicine person for the people.

It is a lot more difficult to be a Native healer today than it was a hundred years ago. The world and the people have changed. There are different kinds of illnesses to deal with now, and not all of them can be attributed to violating the Creator's Natural Laws. There are sicknesses today that are caused by chemical pollution in the environment and our food sources. There are sicknesses caused by stressful living. There are sicknesses caused by poor diet and wrong eating habits. And there are new diseases, injuries, accidents, and mental illnesses being caused by alcohol, tobacco, and drugs. Discrimination, civilization, acculturation, amalgamation, stress, poverty, alcohol and drugs, and poor diet have all wreaked havoc upon our Native people, and a lot of other people in Western society for that matter. The old-time medicine men and women didn't have to deal with these things, though they did have their hands full with new diseases brought on by Western society through measles, smallpox, chicken pox, venereal diseases, tuberculosis, and polio. Today we have cancer, AIDS, prostate gland illnesses, defoliant spray poisoning and mercury poisoning in traditional Native foods, staph infections, strep diseases, cysts on ovaries, skin cancers, allergies, rape, child molestation, diabetes, alcoholism, drug addiction, suicide, family desertion; the list goes on. All of these are a direct result of modern "advancement." Today we have to deal with them as well as with the typical problems of spider bites, injuries, ghosts, evil spirits, sorcery, and taboos.

It takes time for a medicine person to diagnose, study, and learn how to cure new diseases and illnesses. We do not have modern scientific equipment, a research team, or labs and hospitals available to help. We do not receive grants to conduct medical research and come up with new medicines. We use our own meager income to travel and get good, clean herbs, which are now difficult to find. We learn how to diagnose and heal people by becoming ill and injured ourselves; and by learning how to heal ourselves we learn how to heal others with similar problems. We are not allowed to experiment upon our relations in Nature, or on other human beings. There are no established sets of textbooks handed down from one generation to the next that can aid us in our profession. We are not educated in the way of Western physicians, psychiatrists, and psychologists through formal academic preparation, training in the field, experimentation upon patients, exploratory surgery, and pill pushing. We are taught to use our dreams, visions, powers of the earth, personal power, and the Great Creator's power to heal others. We are not always successful because we must continually keep up our own study, growth, learning, development, and profession while trying to raise and support a family. There is no substitute when a medicine man or woman gets sick; you cannot call a backup because there aren't many medicine people around anymore in Indian country, and the remaining few live far apart. It is not like it was in the old days when medicine people teamed up to help a patient, or they could call upon a substitute. So the White doctor gets a lot of our referrals today.

To make matters worse, intermarriage with other races and tribes has compounded the problem and workload. Now we have White, Black, and Yellow people coming to us for doctoring, teaching, ceremony, and wanting to learn "spiritual ways." Most of them think a medicine man or woman is supposed to doctor free of charge or for a minimal donation. It is true that most Native medicine men and women do not charge for their services, but according to custom and tradition some kind of decent donation or payment of respect was given; a healer cannot feed a family on donations of eagle feathers and tobacco, nor afford to gather herbs, pay for the price of wood for sweat lodge ceremonies, or buy doctoring material without money.

Ironic as it may seem, more and more non-Indian people are seeking the Native healer while the Indian people are going to the White doctors. A good medicine man or woman will try to help anyone, regardless of color, race, sex, age, religion, or income, because that is what the Great Creator expects. Most medicine people are highly sensitive, sympathetic, and caring. They take pride in their knowledge and abilities and their profession. They have a lot of love in their hearts for their fellows, for all of creation, and for the Great Creator. Because of this love, it is difficult for medicine people to turn anyone down. They realize that no one can be a healer or serve as a medium between humans, the spirits and the Great Spirit if they are full of anger and hate. Native healers take on the pain, the suffering, and often the illness of the patient. In order to doctor and use the fullest power, they must abstain from sex and social activity; sometimes a healer must also fast, without food or water, as a means to muster stronger power.

There have been a number of occasions where I had to "stay clean" for periods ranging from three days to three weeks in order to help a patient. And there were times I had to fast, pray in the sweat lodge, hike a long way to a certain mountain, and seek a dream or vision in order to get the knowledge or power to heal a particular person. The average doctoring session lasts from two hours to four days. Sometimes, what at first may appear to be a simple case can turn out to be very complex. A medicine person must therefore be committed to seeing the healing through to the end, no matter what it takes.

In this respect you might say that good Native healers go beyond the call of duty in the treatment of patients. They take a holistic approach to doctoring. For example, if the patient complains of a torn tendon, the medicine man or woman will work on the physical injury, but in addition doctor the patient's mind, emotions, and soul. Sometimes the patient's family is directly involved in the healing ceremony, and the patient is always directly involved in his or her own doctoring. The patient is not considered simply an object to be treated but as a fellow human being who is suffering and needs help. The healer has sympathy for the patient because he or she may have suffered a similar injury. So being a medicine man or woman requires patience, understanding, and compassion.

I can share a number of examples with you of how Native healers function in contemporary society. As I said earlier, good Native healers know their own strengths and weaknesses. Well, sometimes an illness or problem might be caused by Western society, its pollution or stressful influence. In such cases the medicine man or woman might not be able to provide the primary care and will encourage the patient to seek medical services from a Western doctor. In this kind of situation, however, the Native healer can provide spiritual and cultural support.

For example, one time my wife had to go into the hospital for major surgery because she was constantly having abdominal pains and some minor bleeding from adhesions. She was afraid of the operation and had a bad dream that she might not live through it. As a result, we asked Billy Mesa, a medicine man, to help doctor her in preparation for the surgery, while she was being operated on, and after the surgery to enhance the healing process. According to Native custom and law we offered him cultural gifts and a money donation to cover his travel expenses and time.

We also got permission from the White surgeon and his medical team to perform a healing ceremony in the hospital room. This can be difficult because most White doctors, nurses, and hospital staff have not been educated about Native American religion, beliefs, and ceremonies. There is the problem of hospital rules, the danger of oxygen, cleanliness, privacy, and sometimes downright prejudice against Indians. So we had to do a lot of appealing, teaching, and negotiating in order to carry out our rights.

The Native healer made four tobacco ties from four different colors of cloth (white, red, yellow, and black), representing the four sacred directions of the Universe. He made an altar of the bed by tying the tobacco prayer offerings to its four corners. He burned cedar in a small stone bowl as a means to purify the patient and the room and to make "protective" medicine upon the patient and her environment. The cedar keeps away bad spirits, deceased people or ghosts who might be wandering around the hospital, curses, and challengers. He smoked his sacred pipe and talked to the Great Creator about the patient's problem and requested spiritual assistance to help calm her state of anxiety, to protect her so she would live through the operation, and he called in his own spirit powers. Afterwards he sang a number of power songs and used some sacred quartz crystals to form a shield of protection of high spiritual light around the patient and her physician. The tobacco ties and crystals were allowed to go into surgery with the patient.

As my wife underwent surgery, the Native healer continued to pray in the hospital room and periodically outside in the courtyard. He studied the different signs and omens. At one point he came into the room and said that he saw a bad sign, a small hawk, and as a result he believed the patient was having complications. So he made his prayers stronger, and engaged the family in prayer and song. All involved were told to hold an image of the patient in mind and focus strong healing energy and protection going into her.

We later found out that the patient had hemorrhaged during surgery and the situation was pretty serious for a while, but the patient was saved due to the medical team's quick response and competency. After surgery the patient was brought to her room for rest and recovery. While she slept the Native healer continued to sing and pray on her. He burned sweetgrass as an offering to his spirits and regalia, he used an eagle wing fan to clean her aura of negative energy, and he used water and the healing power in his hands to doctor the patient's mind, body, and soul (something like "laying on of the hands"). He stayed with the patient for several days, going back to our house periodically to rest.

The healer had already spiritually prepared the home environment when the patient got home from the hospital. The house had been thoroughly smoked up with sage and cedar for protection and purification, and certain power objects such as hawk feathers, tobacco ties, animal hides, and other forms of regalia had been strategically placed around. Symbolically and spiritually these powers were being used for further healing. Then the healer conducted a sacred sweat lodge ceremony involving family and friends, to finalize the healing.

I have known other cases where Native healers, including my wife or myself, were asked to help people in the hospital, in prison, and in convalescent homes. Sometimes the patients were little children, pregnant women, elders, and even people of different races such as Vietnamese, Hispanic, Black, or White. It is more difficult to justify our services to White people because of the hassle we get from White staff and administrators, but occasionally you will find an open-minded authority or physician who is willing to do whatever is necessary to help a patient.

I have personally assisted some of my mentors perform healing on patients who had heart attacks, strokes, cancer, leukemia, auto accidents, work related injuries, gunshot wounds, knife wounds, and mental disorders from tormenting spirits or from substance abuse. In a large number of cases I have witnessed the patient miraculously healed. In a couple of cases I painfully watched patients die because they were too far gone or the Native healer and White doctors just didn't have enough knowledge, power, or skill. Sometimes the patient is not meant to live or really doesn't want to live anymore.

Staying in the hospital for any of the above reasons can be a terrifying experience. The Western medical establishment has a tendency to treat the patient like an object; and as a result the patient often feels lonely, helpless, confused, scared, depressed, or in a state of high anxiety. Mental condition can lower the body's natural immune system or the person's willpower. Thus, according to our Native philosophy and belief, such people should have a healing ceremony done on them to "build up their spirit." In the olden days our Native people had all kinds of rituals to deal with different kinds of experiences, but today, due to the domination of Western society and values, a lot of the Native forms of knowledge and ritualization are not being used. Still, what the Native healer has to offer can prove to be of real value even in a Western-oriented situation.

For example, we have the concept of spiritual, emotional, cultural, and symbolic support for a patient in a hospital. It is not important that the Western physician believe in the possibility of Native or spiritual healing. The main concern should be for the patient. Sometimes the patient needs tangible objectives to see in order to believe in the spiritual; such symbols and objectives also help the patient to believe in himself or herself during a time of weakness and crisis. Under P.L. 95-341, The American Indian Religious Freedom Act, the Native people have a right to this kind of support system and ceremony; under basic human rights, all humans should have the right to some kind of spiritual support system.

There have been a number of occasions when we have helped our non-Native friends, either directly by providing a Native healing ceremony or by teaching them certain forms of practice they could safely use themselves. Examples are how to pray with cedar or sage to protect the patient, how to use quartz crystals to put up a protective shield around the patient, how to visualize healing the patient with mental-spiritual light and energy, and how to pray to the Great Creator, Mother Earth, and good spirits for assistance. We are all the Great Creator's property, and though not many people know it, even White people originally used crystals and herbs in healing ceremonies similar to our Native way; some still do. Hence there are various forms of shamanistic knowledge non-Native people can use without offending the Native religion and beliefs.

My wife and I once performed some healing sessions on Native men who were in a Fairbanks, Alaska, correctional facility. Several of them asked what kind of Native medicine they could use to protect themselves from getting molested or beaten up, and they wanted to know what they could use during times of need in healing. Due to organizational rules they were not allowed to keep herbs and power objects, nor any kind of Native regalia. This is what I told them:

"My brothers, look around you. Even though you are cooped up in this Whiteman's prison you are not alone. The Great Spirit can go through walls and steel, and the powers of Nature He created are at close range. Do not most of you smoke? Our people have always used tobacco as an offering to the Great Creator, our ancestors, to the good spirits, and to our relations in Nature as payment for assistance. Everything in our Universe can be a source of power if only you know how to use it. During the day we have the Grandfather Sun; surely you can see him out your window. At night we have the Grandmother Moon and star people. Even the clouds that pass over this building can help you if you appeal to them. And how many times have you seen the raven come here just before we walked into the building? A number of you commented about it, wondering if it was a coincidence. Even this little spider now dangling down from the ceiling is your relation; she too can help, for she has special powers. You are never alone.

"Even if you don't smoke, try praying with a cigarette; it is allowed in this building. Believe in your ancestors, their cultural knowledge, and your Native ways. Believe with all your heart that things we see in Nature are not simply clouds, birds, Sun or Moon, wind or rain, but they are also spirit powers, for they are. Ask them for help, talk to them about your problems, and help pray for each other. Now try this as an experiment:

"You see this water in this cup? The water is the fourth power of Creation. It is sacred and holy. It is connected to the Great Creator. Nothing can hurt the power and spirit of the water. Think of all the terrible things people do to the water. They holler at it, cuss at it, urinate in it, menstruating women bathe in it, we even bathe deceased people in it. We shoot at it and even throw it in fire! The worst poisons, toxins, germs, diseases, and viruses in the world live in, around, or near the water. The biggest, meanest, most vicious, and deadliest creatures in the world—seen and unseen—live in, around, or near the water. But none of these things can harm the spirit of the water because it purifies itself, it heals itself, and it protects itself. And when the Great Creator wants to purify, protect, or heal the earth does He not use the Spirit of the Water?

"So I am going to share this ancient form of knowledge with you. Remember it and use it. Pray to the Great Creator and the spirit of the water to help you. Every time you drink it, every time you bathe in it, say the prayer I share with you, and you will be helped. And when you finally come out of this terrible place you call the joint, go through a sacred sweat lodge ceremony and use the water and natural powers of Nature to purify you from the violations you committed and the bad experience you had in here."

prayer for purification

O sacred water, the Great Creator put you here on the Earth from the very Beginning of Time to be a healer and purifier. As I understand it, you are both physical and spiritual. The worst poisons, pollution, germs, and diseases in the world live in, around, or near the water. The biggest, meanest, deadliest, and most vicious creatures—seen and unseen—live in and around the water. Still, the water purifies itself. So nothing can harm or hurt you because you purify yourself, protect yourself, and heal yourself. This I ask for your spirit, and I ask for your help and that you doctor me. And I give you thanks for the use of your power.

EPILOGUE

▼   ▼   ▼   ▼   ▼   ▼

I HAVE BEEN ON JUST ABOUT EVERY INDIAN RESERVATION IN the United States. I have also been in a number of Native villages in Alaska, and in numerous urban Indian areas one time or another. I have been to these places for specific reasons: sometimes to do ceremonies, sometimes to perform healing, sometimes to conduct lectures and training workshops, and at other times just to listen and learn.

I hear people say that poverty, unemployment, lack of education, and alcohol is killing off the Native American. These things are, indeed, slowly destroying our people. But the real problem, as I see it, is a loss of spirituality and self-esteem.

At one time our tribes were strong with traditional ceremonies, sacred dances, ancient rituals, and medicine. We must somehow try to recapture and use these forms of power that the Great Creator gave us in the Beginning, if we are going to survive as a species. We must regain our spiritual strength, pride, and dignity and use it to start healing ourselves, our families, and our communities, along with the Mother Earth who also needs healing.

We must learn to be proud of our rich heritage and culture, our tribal religions, our true spiritual knowledge; we should no longer be ashamed of it. And we should not be afraid to share it with each other as was done in the olden days. Despite our differences in language, religion, beliefs, and practices, as Native people we all have one common bond—our ancient and direct connection with the true Great Creator of the Universe.

Our tribal medicines, our power centers upon this earth, our ancient ceremonies, and our spiritual forms of knowledge cry out to be used; and we should use these things with sincerity and respect. Thus, I hope the information in this book can be used for that purpose and not unjustly criticized as a simple romanticism or commercialization of Native religion. I hope it can serve to teach those who want to learn how to "reconnect" with their Creator, their spirit, the Mother Earth, and each other.

APPENDIX

spiritual violations

▼   ▼   ▼   ▼   ▼   ▼

1. Human beings are not supposed to have sex in Nature; upon the mountains, in the woods, on the desert, in meadows, on or near the ocean, nor in creeks, lakes, and rivers. *Reason:* Such places are the residence of good and bad spirits, they do not like to be contaminated by "human's" smell and activity.

2. It is against the law to molest, kill, or experiment upon animals, birds, snakes, bugs, trees, plants, fish, and human beings needlessly. *Reason:* Such entities are the Great Creator's property. They

have been placed on Earth for a purpose and function. Humankind does not have the right or authority to destroy or molest the Creator's property without just cause and restitution.

3. It is against the Creator's Law for menstruating women to walk, hike, swim, or bathe in Nature, or have sex while on their menses. *Reason:* Nature is purifying the women mentally, physically, and spiritually. As a consequence, toxins and negative energy are being discharged and it can contaminate others and Nature. By the same token the women are being replenished with positive spiritual power. She should therefore isolate herself, purify herself, center herself with the cosmic forces, rejuvenate herself; and not disperse her powers socially, physically, mentally, or spiritually.

4. It is against the Creator's Law for humans to have unusual sex acts. *Reason:* Humans were originally "souls" at one time. They broke the Creator's Law when they left the spirit world and took over the bodies of animals in order to experience sex. Humans are expected to be humanlike and develop their soul toward spiritual purity. Thus animal type sex acts are considered impure and unnatural for humans. Violation of this law can cause mental, physical, and spiritual sickness.

5. It is against the Creator's Law to murder, rape, torture, or commit suicide. *Reason:* Human beings are the property of the Great Creator and therefore sacred. Humankind does not have the right or authority to abuse the Great Creator's property.

6. Human beings are not supposed to participate in prayer, sacred ceremonies, rituals, or healing while under the influence of alcohol, sex, or menses. *Reason:* Spiritual power is pure and must therefore be treated with respect, purity, and clarity.

7. It is against the Creator's Law to use witchcraft or to make bad prayers, bad thoughts, bad wishes, or use evil power against others. *Reason:* The Great Creator made everything in the Universe including human beings and powers. He established law and order amongst the created. The first Law of the Land was respect for all living things, including the Earth, Universe, and humankind. The use of evilness abridges the law of respect and causes harm to others.

8. Human beings must always be "clean" whenever they hunt, fish, or gather herbs. This means a clean body, no sex, no alcohol, nor women on their menses. *Reason:* Natural foods and plants have power. Human beings should always "pray" to the entity before taking its life and explain why it is being used. Humans must be clean mentally, physically, and spiritually whenever praying and using this power. In this way the spiritual powers of the entity will be transferred to the human along with the physical properties. Nature's powers strengthen our soul and enrich our health. Negative powers contaminate our soul and weaken our health. Abuse of "powers" causes sickness to the violator.

9. Human beings should not waste their life on

drugs, alcohol, selfishness, or idleness. *Reason:* Every human being was placed on this earth for a purpose and reason. The Creator wants all human beings to discover their purpose in life and carry out their function. Humans are sacred and should therefore not waste their life. To do so will cause sickness, natural life will shorten, death may occur.

(This list is used by Native healers in northwest California.)

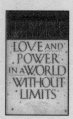
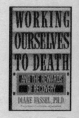
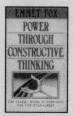

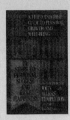

THE TEMPLETON PLAN

From one of Wall Street's wisest investors comes a tried and true guide to personal growth and well-being. By following John Templeton's 21-step program — one step a day for three weeks — vital, connnections between beliefs in religious principles and belief in yourself are revealed, enabling you to become a successful and happy person.

IF ONLY HE KNEW

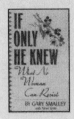

Gary Smalley explains a woman's deepest needs, shows a man how to meet those needs, and gives ten simple steps to strengthen any marriage. He helps men to understand not only how to respond to a woman's feelings, but also how to make her feel important. This invaluable guide filled with case histories and biblical examples maps a blueprint to a better marriage for today's modern man.

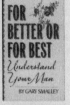

FOR BETTER OR FOR BEST

What motivates men and what natural qualities do women use to build a better marriage? In the tradition of Deborah Tannen's bestselling *You Just Don't Understand,* Gary Smalley helps women to understand not only the way men think, but also how to move a man's heart. With empathy, humor, and wisdom, Smalley solves every practical and emotional problem a woman can face in her marriage.